rescue your nails

a do-it-yourself guide to perfect fingers & toes

rescue your nails

a do-it-yourself guide to perfect fingers & toes

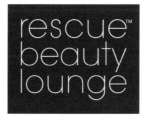

rescue™
beauty
lounge

by Ji Baek

workman publishing · new york

This book is for everyone who's stepped in and out of life
at Rescue Beauty Lounge . . . but especially to my daily sunshine,
my most loving husband, partner, and best friend, Alex.
Without your love, patience, support, and dedication,
Rescue Beauty Lounge wouldn't be here.

Copyright © 2008 by Ji Baek

Library of Congress Cataloging-in-Publication Data

Baek, Ji.
Rescue your nails : a do-it-yourself guide to perfect fingers & toes / Ji Baek.
    p. cm.
Includes bibliographical references and index.
ISBN 978-0-7611-4377-2 (alk. paper)
1. Nails (Anatomy)—Care and hygiene. 2. Manicuring. 3. Beauty, Personal. I. Title.
RL94.B325 2007
646.7'27—dc22   2007024000

Cover design by Janet Parker
Book design by Janet Parker with Carrie Hamilton
Principal photography by Deborah Ory and Jenna Bascom

Workman books are available at special discounts when purchased in bulk for premiums and sales promotions as well as for fund-raising or educational use. Special editions or book excerpts can also be created to specification. For details, contact the Special Sales Director at the address below.

Workman Publishing Company, Inc.
225 Varick Street
New York, NY 10014-4381
www.workman.com

Printed in the United States of America
First printing April 2008

10 9 8 7 6 5 4 3 2 1

thank you, thank you

It took a lot of people to turn this book into a reality. Nina Reznick, without your intelligence and guidance this book couldn't exist. I'm so grateful to David Kirsch for sending you into my life. I'm truly blessed to have you as a friend, confidant, and brilliant agent/lawyer. This world benefits from your endless passion, dedication, and generosity. Thanks also to the amazing team at Workman Publishing, especially Peter Workman, Suzanne Rafer, Helen Rosner, Janet Parker, and everyone that worked so extremely hard for this book—I'm forever grateful.

Since we opened Rescue Beauty Lounge in 1998, we've been extremely lucky to have generous support from the media—publications local, national, and international, not to mention television and the Internet. A million thanks to all the directors, editors, writers, journalists, reporters, producers, freelancers, assistants, interns, and whoever has ever been involved in the process of getting the Rescue name out there. Truly my gratitude is endless. All my clients whom I know and love, you have enriched my life. Working with you has been a fabulous journey! Thank you so much for being part of the Rescue Beauty Lounge family! I cherish your gorgeous support.

Over the years, Alex and I have always been incredibly proud of all the staff and technicians who have come through our door. The biggest joy we take from our company is guiding, teaching, training—and learning from—our staff. We take pride in all of you, and think you—and all nail and beauty technicians everywhere—are deserving of tremendous appreciation. Of course, to our current staff, thank you so much for all your hard work. Let's keep it up!

To my beautiful circle of friends and family: Your heart, ears, and shoulders are precious and priceless. Especially my adoring mom—without your wisdom, unconditional love, and your endless prayers, I might not be the person that I am today.

This book is in loving memory of Raisa Sobolevsky—avid reader, magical gardener, and never an "in-law," but a second mother. I miss you so deeply. And to my daddy: I may not have followed the map of life you had laid out for me, but I can feel and know that you are all smiles up there. I love you and miss you. You are always in my heart.

contents

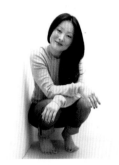

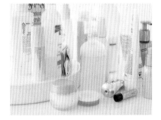

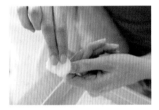

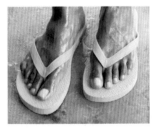

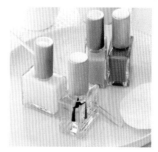

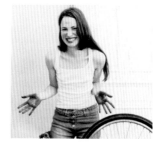

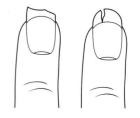

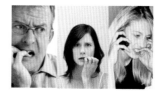

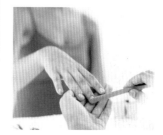

INTRODUCTION

rescue to the rescue

I can tell everything I need to know about you by looking at your nails.

Did you just take a quick, nervous look at your hands? Relax! You don't have to bury them deep in your pockets. This book will show you how to make your nails look their best. Trust me, once you feel good about your nails, the rest of your life will fall right into place. Nail care has a lot to teach us, but for now, let's focus on three absolutes:

- Nothing has to be complicated.
- Everything is fixable.
- A little bit of TLC goes a long way.

I have an "extreme makeover" client who is no stranger to personal care—her face is pulled back tight, her lips so bee-stung that they're almost clownlike, her hair layered with blond highlights, and her body swathed in designer clothing. After her manicure one day, I examined her hands, admiring the job her technician had done. She interrupted my inspection, stating, "You know, I absolutely loathe the way this polish looks!"

"Let's take it off and change it to something else!" I responded. She looked surprised, and I could tell she was thinking "Is it that simple? So easy? That's it?"

Yes—it *is* that simple, even in the complex world in which we live. Unlike many other beauty treatments, nail care is about instant gratification and looking good—with no complications. You have to wait for a bad haircut or dye job to grow out, or see a doctor if you have second thoughts about your plastic surgery or Botox. Nails, though, are something you can change easily—color can be applied or removed in minutes; the length can be changed on a whim. No matter the state of your hair, the shape of your body, or the condition of your clothes, your nails can (and will) look terrific. A good manicure, like a good haircut, has an amazing effect on your self-confidence. It's *the* instant pick-me-up.

Unlike a haircut, you can do a manicure yourself—at home—without spending a fortune on fancy creams and polishes or going to the germ-ridden corner nail spa (more on that later). Taking care of your nails should be an enjoyable ritual, not a chore.

Grooming sessions allow you time to chat with your girlfriends, bond with your loved ones, or just spend some quiet meditative time alone. Whether it's an hour-long salon pedicure, an at-home soak, or just a simple buffing, the step-by-step instructions in this book will help take the mystery out of the manicure.

The importance of a manicure is much, much more than just the coat of polish at the end. In chapter 1, I'll tell you a little bit about my background in the nail care industry, and about the history of the industry as a whole. In chapter 2, we'll go through what's in your medicine cabinet (and what *should* be there), demystifying products and packaging so that at-home nail care is as simple and straightforward as taking care of your skin or hair. In chapters 3 and 4, I'll share my tried-and-true tips for doing your own manicures and pedicures—from soaking and scrubbing through cuticle care and filing. And of course, the icing on the cake: Chapter 5 brings us back to the beautiful, with detailed breakdowns of polish colors and a no-fail technique for flawless self-polishing.

Of course, it's not all basic nail care. Chapter 6 gives you the inside scoop on caring for your hands to help offset the effects of aging, environmental exposure, and harsh working conditions—including the office. And then there's the ugly stuff: Chapter 7 has straight talk on dealing with hangnails, split nails, calluses, and other bits of unpleasantness. My famous nail-biting cure, NBA (Nail-Biters Anonymous), is outlined in Chapter 8.

Finally, for those days when you're feeling especially luxurious, chapter 9 brings it into the salon: etiquette, germ awareness, and what to expect when you turn the care of your hands and feet over to a professional nail technician. Of course, with everything you'll learn from all the chapters that come before, you'll be the next best thing to a professional yourself. But as much fun as it can be to do your own nails, let's be honest—we all deserve a little splurge sometimes!

Throughout the book you'll notice that I draw a hard line about some things: the importance of moisturization, the necessity of using sterile tools, commitment to keeping your hands protected in every environment. If you want flawless, hand-model-quality hands and nails, follow my instructions to a T. One look at my hands will tell a different story, though: I've worked with my hands all my life, and sometimes it's just not possible to keep up a moisturization routine *plus* wearing gloves *plus* avoiding cuts and scrapes *plus* this and that and the other thing. Use my tips as guidelines, not laws. The most important thing isn't that your fingers and toes be as flawless as a hand model's—it's that they suit you and your life.

At my Rescue Beauty
Lounge in New York's
Meatpacking District—
the center of it all.

you've got nail

Regardless of how attentive we are to it, some kind of nail care is a regular part of all of our lives. In fact, taking care of our nails is one of the first beauty treatments we're taught. We trim them, file them, or bite them off. And for some of us, nail care can also be frivolous and fun—we paint our fingers and toes in colors tasteful or tacky, or buff and groom them and let them go naked. You can tell a lot about people by how they take care of their nails.

Nails fascinate me now, but my life hasn't always been about them. In fact, if you had told me twenty years ago that one day I would become a top nail care expert, I would have laughed.

I never had nice nails when I was growing up; I wasn't allowed to. I grew up in South Korea in the 1970s, where my very traditional mother set me on the path to becoming a concert pianist. There was no negotiation when it came to piano practice: Long nails were forbidden—it's impossible to play properly with them. Nail polish? Never! That was only for trashy little girls; it was as bad as wearing makeup! I remember begging for little pearly seashell pink dots of nail polish on my tiny, tiny nails, but the response was always a firm no.

My childhood experience with nail color was limited to an ancient ritual handed down from my grandmother to my mother, and eventually to my sisters and me. As the ladies of the Korean royal court had done for hundreds of years, the three generations of women in my family would gather to celebrate the summer solstice. My grandmother and my mother would

As our nails grew out

and the half-moon stain slowly disappeared from our fingertips, we knew summer was coming to an end.

crush special red flower petals called *bong sung wha*, which they would then mix with a secret powder to make a paste. We would apply the red paste to our hands, wrap our nails in the flower's leaves, and cover the leaves with plastic tied with thread. We would leave the wrappings on all night, and in the morning we would peel them away to reveal our red-stained fingers. The color would wash off of our skin in a day or two, leaving a deep geranium-orange stain on our fingernails.

As our nails grew out and the half-moon stain slowly disappeared from our fingertips, we knew summer was coming to an end. My mother and grandmother loved this ancient ritual that connected our family to the noble ladies of old Korea. But I thought the stain was a poor substitute for the slick, shiny nail polish I wanted.

Land of Opportunity

We moved to America when I was 12, and I thought my luck would change. It didn't. The only thing that did change was that I couldn't understand what anyone was talking about—I didn't speak a word of English. Still, I was fascinated by the American culture that surrounded me: women with blond hair and blue eyes, living dolls like the Barbies that my dad would bring back to Korea from his trips to Paris. And television! My mother believed that *Sesame Street* was an ideal way to learn English, but I had other plans. Soon I was clicking through all the forbidden channels, that is, anything with commercials, anything *but* PBS. I embraced it all: longing for that Jordache look while simultaneously watching Brooke Shields advertise Calvin Klein jeans. I wanted to try every cereal under the sun, the more artificially colored the better. I longed for feathered hair, tight jeans, caked-on eyeshadow, purple mascara, and an endless supply of grape-flavored Bonne Bell lip gloss. I was ready to be an American teenager—long, neon-painted nails and all.

Once we moved to our new home, my mother switched me from the very solitary piano to the slightly more social viola. Her thought was that being part of an orchestra would make me more connected with disciplined "classical music people," and save me from the evil American culture that she feared was ruining her innocent daughter. It almost worked: Yes, I diligently practiced my music, but I also danced around lip-synching "Like a Virgin."

I might have had a viola case in my hand, but I was the height of trendy in my lace leggings, orange Converse high-tops covered with my own graffiti, a neon-bright oversize shirt, Ray-Bans, and twenty-two black rubber bracelets stacked up my arm (I counted them every day). I went around blasting Madonna and Depeche Mode on my Walkman, the viola case my most unfashionable accessory.

But I *still* couldn't have the long nails that were the height of fashion in the eighties. Well, that's not entirely true. I could have four of them: the four fingers that held the bow; all the others still had to be short. What was I going to do with four long nails? Nothing. I spent my teenage years longing for the day when I would be free to do whatever I wanted with my nails.

But be careful what you wish for! In college I majored in music, but just as things started to take off, I began to suffer from tendinitis. Eventually the pain became so intense that I was forced to give up playing musical instruments entirely, and my life was turned upside down. It was strange and scary—suddenly, having

> I spent my teenage years longing for the day when I would be free to do whatever I wanted with my nails.

The History of Nails

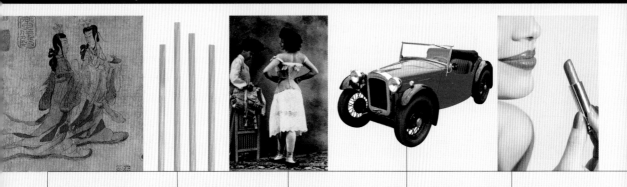

3000 BC: Chinese aristocrats color their nails with a lacquer made of beeswax and egg whites dyed with plants and metals. Red and black are reserved for the highest levels of royalty. Peasants found coloring their nails could be put to death.

1830: In France, Dr. Sitts, podiatrist to King Louis Philippe, advocates gentle nail care with a tool made of orangewood. In 1892 his method is introduced to women—the first modern manicure.

1899: In her book *A Complete and Authentic Treatise on the Laws of Health and Beauty,* Harriet Hubbard Ayer advises against too-tight corsets, warning that they lead to unattractively red hands.

1925: French makeup artist Michelle Ménard introduces dye-based fingernail polish. Its chemical composition is inspired by automobile paint.

1932: Brothers Charles and Joseph Revson, founders of Revlon, develop pigment-based polish, enabling the fashion of matching your fingernails to your lipstick.

long nails and being fashionable were the last things on my mind, as I pined for the life that I no longer had. I forgot how much I had hated the structure and discipline of music study, and wished that I could be exactly the kind of person that I had so violently fought against becoming.

After music performance stopped being the center of my life, I shifted my focus to something new: the restaurant industry. After college I threw myself into it full force, attracted to the unexpected similarities between a well-run restaurant and a well-run orchestra: All the pieces need to work together in harmony, requiring both talent and discipline. I took a position as a front-of-house manager at a loud, busy, hip restaurant in Manhattan.

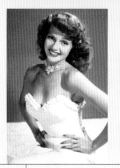 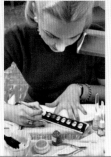 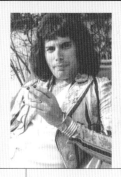 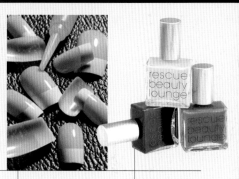

1940: Rita Hayworth popularizes long, oval, fiery-red nails as the ultimate sex symbol.

1950: The nail stencil is patented, and becomes a popular way to ensure a perfect polish application— no coloring outside the lines!

1975: In an interview with *Circus* magazine, gender-bending rock star Freddie Mercury says of his infamous nail polish, "Black seems to be the color for me."

1980s: The French manicure, a nude base with white tips, is the epitome of chic. Women buy press-on nails to get the look at home.

2008 and beyond: Anything goes! From bright primary yellow to palest whisper pink, the chicest nails are short, well-groomed, and clad in virtually every color of the rainbow.

I stomped and clicked through the early nineties, asserting my authority, wearing four-inch heels (as a small woman in the loud, aggressive, male-dominated restaurant world, I needed all the height I could get). I was far too busy running around the restaurant floor and shouting orders to have time for any sort of self-maintenance: I kept buying new clothes and underwear to avoid washing my clothes, and just ignored my aching feet. But eventually I turned to logical, practical solutions: I discovered drop-off laundry service, and pedicures for my poor toes.

I was attracted to the word itself. *Pedicure:* Cure your feet. I really was in dire need; my poor dogs were barking incessantly. And the attention they got? It was worth every penny. I was also

"Are you there, God?

It's me, Ji.
Isn't there a
clean place
to get a pedicure
in this town?"

a little shocked—that pedicure really made my toes beautiful! I remember coming home at four in the morning after a late shift at the restaurant and standing in the shower, just staring in awe at my toes, candy red and perfect. I realized at that moment the real importance of nail care: It's not for looking pretty, or for showing off, or for impressing a potential mate. You need to do it for yourself. I resolved to get pedicures regularly.

My new pedicure addiction gave me two choices. I could go to the corner salons that stud Manhattan, where you walk in, cross your fingers, and hope for the best. Or I could get my pedicures at a big, super-expensive place that offers a hair salon and spa services. But beyond differences in price and décor, both types shared the same ingredients. They both seemed dirty (mysterious portable footbaths and fancy whirlpools were deeply disturbing to my germaphobic nature—years of working in a restaurant had instilled in me a preternatural loathing for cross-contamination), and both lacked a good concept of service or marketing. After a while, I started feeling desperate—*Are you there, God? It's me, Ji. Isn't there a clean place to get a pedicure in this town?*

I left the high-stress restaurant world soon after getting married, and I quickly grew bored with being a full-time "domestic goddess." Instead, I directed my energy at my fingers and toes. In my obsessive search for the perfect pedicure, I realized no nail service would live up to my standards—upscale or downscale, nothing felt right to me. They reused the files or the buffing blocks, the technicians were impolite, or the service itself was imperfectly done. I'd always had a strong sense of "If you want something done right, do it yourself," so I turned all that energy toward the nail industry. Soon I was researching small business models and drawing up plans.

My husband questioned my sanity: Did I really want to play right into the tired old stereotype of a Korean woman opening a nail salon? But after I pitched my business plan to him, he came around to the idea, and I enrolled in beauty school to get my technician's license.

The idea for Rescue Beauty Lounge came to me one day in Paris. I had accompanied my husband on one of his business trips, and I found myself sitting at a café by myself on one of those perfect dove-gray November afternoons. I always carry a notebook with me, and I was jotting down my ideas for my as yet unnamed nail spa. I knew I wanted to correct the flaws I had seen in other spas: I wanted my tools to be sterilized in an autoclave (more about that on page 155), the technicians to wear gloves, the service to include high-quality products (none of that mysterious pink lotion in an unmarked bottle), clients to be treated in private rooms where they could relax, unwind, luxuriate—and bring their friends.

Most important—I wanted to train the staff myself. As I sat there, my mind wandered, and I thought about the path my life had taken: from a disciplined child musician to a harried restaurant manager to a perfection-oriented housewife. I realized that what I wanted was just to be taken away from it all. I wanted to be rescued, and so I wrote it down: Rescue Beauty Lounge.

True to its name, Rescue saved me. It saved me and ten years later it's still going strong—every day it saves the women and men (yes, men!) who come here looking for a solution to their nail-grooming problems. They find a clean, relaxed environment for nail care, not an anonymous chop shop, where they can get a pick-me-up or an update on the latest trends. Think of this book as a little piece of Rescue in your home.

> What I wanted was just to be taken away from it all. I wanted to be rescued.

The Evolution of Beautiful Nails

Does "perfect" really exist? I'm not sure about any other category in life, but when it comes to nails, yes. Yes, perfect does exist. But you have to be willing to work for it.

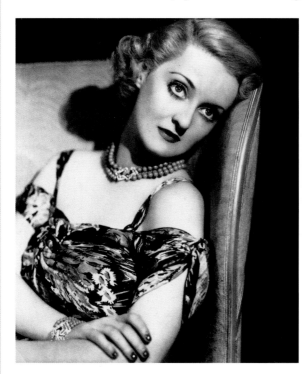

Bette Davis: the consummate hand model.

Our notion of the perfect set of nails has evolved over time. The ideal style changes from generation to generation, and you can often see it in an intergenerational gathering of women: long 1950s-style nails on a grandmother, the midlength French manicure of the power-suit '90s on a mother, and brooding black purple on the fingers of a fashion-conscious teenage daughter. Many women adopt the nail style of their heyday and then stick to it, with loyalties to particular polish colors and nail care brands that are as fierce as the loyalties that build to cult-classic face creams.

But no matter what era your nails reflect, there's beauty to be found. The flawless claws on Bette Davis in *All About Eve* are perfectly evocative of the 1940s and '50s (I still get goose bumps whenever I see her take a drag on that cigarette), and you might remember your grandmother or your mother sitting at the kitchen table, lovingly tending to her own Bette Davis set, maybe lamenting having broken a nail that week.

Almost in direct response to the high-maintenance look of the 1950s, the '60s saw a return to natural nails: polish-free and short. This was right in tune with the anti-beauty-enhancement movement of that era: long, unadorned hair and natural, makeup-free faces, reflecting the bra-burning back-to-nature notion that permeated the era. But the pendulum swung again: Advances in nail polish formulas brought pearlescent and metallic shades onto the market, and the seventies saw frosty, shiny colors on the grooviest fingernails—a trend that lasted through the decade.

The early eighties were the era of "think big!" Everyone wanted to look big: big hair, big shoulder pads, floor-length fur coats, chunky jewelry, bright colors, and—the most important part—big nails. Long nails, intricately designed or boldly colored, were in high demand, and impatient consumers who didn't want to sit around waiting for their nails to grow put artificial nails on the map. Silk or linen overlays, while costly, became popular, and when inexpensive acrylic nails became available at salons, the demand for long nails exploded.

This demand for professionally applied artificial nails essentially established the entire nail care industry as we know it. But then came the big scare: Nail fungus was found to thrive underneath artificial nails, and the trendsetters had no choice but to take the false nails off, cut their own nails short, and leave them pale—their nails were so weak that they couldn't hold polish. It was the beginning of an accidental fad: The next generation wore their nails short and pale as well.

By the time Rescue opened in the late nineties, "ghetto fabulous" was the height of style. Hip-hop culture was bursting with energy, and its influence spilled over to everything from makeup to the fashion runway. The pale, short nail look was out, and all the fashion-conscious women flocked to us for long, square nail extensions to go with their hip-hop-inspired look.

Rescue took it one step further: We turned nail art into a mainstream trend. It all started when I painted tiny, tiny daisies all over my toenails in an attempt to add a sweet, pretty side

> Rescue took it **one step further:** We turned nail art into a mainstream trend.

a field guide to the fingernail

If you want to get technical about it, here's what's actually going on at the end of your finger. Each part has its role to play—but don't worry, there won't be a test!

Hyponychium
The point at the tip of your finger at which your nail plate separates from your nail bed. Nail growth past this point is safe to trim.

Nail Plate
The nail itself, made of a translucent protein called keratin.

Lunula
Also known as the "half moon," this whitish curve at the base of the nail is actually part of the matrix: It's made of keratin cells that haven't fully flattened to become the translucent material of the rest of your nail. The curve of the lunula mirrors the natural curve of your nail's edge.

Matrix
The root of the nail, located from the top of the lunula down to a few millimeters past the pterygium. It produces keratin cells, which move up and out as more and more are created. The longer your matrix is, the more cells it will produce, and the thicker your nail will be. Damage to the matrix can mean permanent irregular nail growth—so it's critical that the pterygium and eponychium are working to protect it!

Nail Bed
The extremely sensitive skin beneath the nail plate is a sealed environment that's home to a dense concentration of blood vessels, nerve endings, and melanin-producing cells called melanocytes.

Perionychium
The side edges of the nail plate, where skin overlies the nail by a few millimeters.

Pterygium
The pterygium, or true cuticle, is the fold of thickened skin at the base of the nail plate under which the nail emerges from the matrix.

Eponychium
The thin layer of cuticle that seals the pterygium to the nail plate, protecting the matrix against infection.

to balance out the aggressive shapes and colors of the hip-hop craze. Immediately all our clients begged to have their toes done the same way. I gave in for one beauty editor, and the rest is history. Inspired even further by hip-hop, designer logos made a big comeback. We translated that into nailwear: Our clients studded their nails with hundreds of rhinestones in intricate designs, from Louis Vuitton's interlocking monogram to pink camouflage. We even painted designer fabrics onto toenails! You name it, we did it—and we did it beautifully.

This was an important moment for nails: It was the moment that they became a true accessory. Suddenly designers were requesting specific polish colors for their runway shows, something that had rarely happened before. At last, the fashion elite truly understood that the art and fun of fashion could be extended to nails.

But all good things must come to an end. After September 11, 2001, the economy, and with it the fashion world, took a sharp turn. Fashion and beauty editors would call me to see if it was still "in" to do nail art, or if the somber mood that gripped everyone really extended all the way down to our fingertips. It would have been easy to lie and get more press and more income, but knowing when a trend ends is key—in fashion and beauty, timing is everything. Fashion, politics, and even the economy shape the way we do our nails.

This was an important moment for nails.

However, more than just large-scale factors influence how we do our nails. In the age of working mothers, BlackBerries, iPhones, and text messaging, it's hard to maintain long, beautiful tips. For most women nowadays, the shape of the ideal nail has changed to something a little more practical. There's nothing wrong with having long nails, but today's lifestyle is different from that of women in the Bette Davis golden age, with cigarettes in long holders and a maid to help you dress yourself.

the ten
(UNBREAKABLE)
rules of nail care

1 **Take your vitamins.** Nails are keratin-based, so make sure you have enough calcium, protein, and nutrients in your diet.

2 **Moisturize and hydrate.** Dryness can cause your nails to crack and split. Use moisturizer for your outside, drink plenty of water for your inside.

3 **Keep your nails clean.** There is nothing more unattractive than having dirt under your nails—remember, clean is chic!

4 **File your nails weekly into a smooth,** even shape, whether they're short or long.

5 **Take care of your tools.** Learn the three S's—sterilization, sanitation, and storage—and be vigilant. Preventable infections are just that—preventable!

6 **Trust your instincts.** If it hurts, don't do it. If it feels wrong, stop it. If (heaven forbid) it bleeds, tend to it immediately.

7 **If it chips, take it off!** If you can see the chip, *everyone* can see the chip. Uniformly lovely nails are just a swipe of remover away.

8 **Don't be a slave to trends.** If you're seeing the same color everywhere, only wear it if you like the way it looks. Say no to peer pressure!

9 **Don't be afraid of trends.** Get out of your rut and try something new!

10 **Have fun! Experiment!** Remember, your nails' style is hardly permanent. If you're even slightly tired of your current look, change it! If you're not happy, all it takes is some polish remover and you're back in the safety zone.

But of course, even unbreakable rules were made to be broken!

Today, there is nothing sexier to me than short, round, colored nails: bright reds, dark blood reds, and even crazy colors like black. Can you really pull off wearing black nail polish? Absolutely. It looks great on everyone, no matter what the skin tone or nail shape, as long as the nails are short and even. "Wouldn't it make my fingers look stumpy?" No, but ultimately you're the judge. We each have our own "iconic" idea of how our hands and nails should look.

It seems silly to me that in our pursuit of perfection, we ignore the simple truth: We don't need much more from our nails than that they be healthy, practical to our lifestyle, and beautifully groomed.

You Are Your Nails

Nails can transform your identity, and they are a valuable accessory that helps you send a message. You can make them say whatever you'd like about you: It's easy to use them to help you express a role, a mood, or an identity. Then, after you've made your statement, it's just as easy to change them to reflect a new one.

At Rescue Beauty Lounge, I work with many actors who are preparing for roles. They're often surprised by how much the shape, length, and color of their nails affects the way they inhabit their roles. After sitting down with them for a manicure, without fail, their response is: "Who knew that changing my nails would bring out my character's most revealing gestures?"

One actor client of mine was preparing for a role as a mafioso. I suggested that he come in for a weekly manicure with clear nail polish. He agreed to give my idea a try. A few weeks later, he reported back: "You were absolutely right about this clear polish business. My movements became so pronounced, and I was so much more confident about talking with my hands."

"Who knew that changing my nails would bring out my character's **most revealing** gestures?"

Chapter One

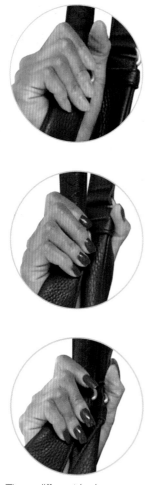

Three different looks,
three different attitudes.

Actresses go through the same thing. One of my clients explained her character to me: a woman of moderate means who was dating a man well above her social class, who felt awkward and out of place at his high-society functions, surrounded by society swans and vast wealth. "She's trying desperately to fit in," said my client. "But her transformation is less than perfect. I need to feel awkward and vulnerable." I knew the answer immediately: nail extensions, with unglamorous French tips about a quarter inch longer than the fashionable length. When we put the extensions on her, the change was immediate. She carried herself differently, walked differently, even changed the way she opened her wallet to get her credit card. Changing her nails changed the way she interacted with the world.

Adopting the right persona through your nails isn't a trick that's restricted to actors and actresses. The job interview is the classic example of when the state of your nails *really* matters. If your career depends on your being questioned and judged by a stranger, do you really want to leave *anything* up to chance?

One of my regular clients was going for an interview at a high-profile fashion magazine. After discussing her outfit, she asked for my advice about nail color. Considering the nature of the position and the people who would be interviewing her, I told her that I didn't really see her going with a color at all, just a beautiful natural buff. We wanted her to be understated but confident, a trendmaker so perfectly groomed that she didn't need color to hide behind. It's what I would have done if I were in her position—and it worked!

When you meet someone new, the way you groom your nails is one of the early giveaways about your personality. Let's visualize a woman wearing a classic white T-shirt, well-fitting jeans, and flip-flops, with her hair in a neat ponytail. She's dressed in a classic casual Saturday afternoon getup—nothing much to tell us anything about her. That is, until we consider the state of her nails. Not even taking into account the concept of color, her nails are a subtle revelation of her character.

Who do you imagine she is if you notice that she has short nails of uneven length, no definite shape, and no polish—not even a buff? Is that the same person whose nails are neatly trimmed to an even length—not too long and not too short—with rounded tips and a coat of shiny polish? What if her nails are artificially long, severely squared at the tip, and coated in glittery lacquer?

I'll leave it to you to draw your own conclusions on who this person is when she's wearing each of her three different sets of nails, but I'd be surprised if you told me you didn't perceive three very different vibes. The wonderful part, of course, is that there's no "right" or "wrong" answer as to which look works best for her—it all depends on what she wants to project about herself.

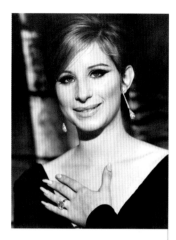

I love Barbra Streisand, and she's the only woman who could pull this off. Plus, it was 1968—don't try this at home!

To that end, when my clients ask me for advice on the length, shape, and color of their nails, I try to be sensitive to what they want their nails to say. This happens all the time in fashion magazines: Editors use the models' nails to subtly reinforce the tone of a fashion shoot. Even wearing the same outfit, with the same hair and makeup, the heroine of one fashion story can sport a natural, short, no-nail-polish look, and come across as an entirely different character from one with nail extensions and black polish.

Ultimately, though, you want to consider the realities of your life when you're deciding what your nails should look like. Don't get me wrong—there's nothing inherently problematic with having long nails, whether they're natural or artificial, but they do require effort to keep up. If you do try to maintain long nails, make sure they are always even! Make a promise to yourself that if one nail breaks, you'll cut them all off and start over again. Your nails grow 3 millimeters a month, on average. Be patient! There is nothing worse than uneven nails!

the real deal on fakes

Though fake nails may make you feel like a diva, they require divalike attention. So before you make a commitment to artificial nails, here are a few things to consider:

■ If your nails are not healthy to begin with, fake nails are only going to make them worse. Hiding bad nails under polish or, in this case, plastic, is not a cure! The chemical binding agents used to affix the fake nails are often harsh and can leave your natural nails brittle and weak, so be sure they're in good shape before attaching the talons.

■ As your natural nails grow, they will become exposed to the air. If any moisture seeps beneath the fake nail, you're putting yourself at risk for a nasty bacterial or fungal infection. So, when your nail tech tells you that—gasp!— you need to come in nearly once a week for a fill-in or touch-up, listen to her!

■ Stay away from swimming pools, lakes, and the ocean. If any moisture,

sand, or dirt gets beneath the artificial nail, I can guarantee you will be faced with some sort of nail-related repercussion. Wear gloves during housecleaning.

■ If your nail technician needs to use a face mask when applying the nails, you do, too!

■ Because of all the filing and sanding as the artificial ones are affixed, your cuticles may sustain some damage. Ask your technician to be as gentle as possible.

■ Because all of the chemical adhesives, the heavy sanding and filing, and the obvious exposure to nail polish and remover that go along with artificial nails, it's best for expectant moms to wait until after they've had their babies to wear fakes, just to be safe.

■ Nail polish lasts far longer on artificial nails than it does on natural ones. While your own nails produce natural oils over the course of the day—which causes them to chip or peel—fakes stay dry, so polish adheres for days and days!

TAKING OFF THE TALONS

Applying artificial nails may seem like a good idea if your nails are less than perfect, but oftentimes weak nails will only become weaker after you remove the fakes.

There is nothing worse for your natural nails than forceful removal of artificial nails. If you don't have time to go to the salon, and you absolutely must take them off at home, be sure to use pure acetone. If you only have acetone-based polish remover, it will still work, but will take twice as long.

At-Home Artificial Nail Removal

You'll need:

Nail scissors or clippers	A white buffing block or disk
A medium- or coarse-grained nail file	Wooden orange stick or sterilized cuticle pusher
A small bowl	Towels (paper or cloth)
Pure acetone or acetone-based nail polish remover	Moisturizer

1. Using the clippers or scissors, trim your artificial nails until they aren't much longer than your natural nails—the shorter they are, the easier they are to remove. The nail shouldn't extend past your fingertip.

2. Even out the surface of the artificial nail: With your medium- or coarse-grained file, gently file down any caked-on dried glue, acrylic, or gel.

3. Soak your fingers for 2 to 3 minutes in a bowl filled with acetone or nail polish remover.

4. Remove your hand from the acetone and gently buff down the surface of the nail with your white buffing block. Re-soak and re-buff until the artificial nail has completely dissolved.

5. If the artificial nail starts to lift from your natural nail, you can use a clean orange stick or a sterilized metal cuticle pusher to help it along, but be gentle!

6. Rinse your hands thoroughly with soap and warm water, and dry them gently.

7. Inspect your nails and buff away any residual glue, acrylic, or gel. Wash one more time, and finish off with moisturizer!

After you've removed the artificial nails, your natural ones will probably be weak and brittle. The best thing to do to jump-start nail growth after fakes is to give yourself a manicure (see The At-Home Rescue Manicure, page 39) or head to the salon for a professional one. Be sure to keep your nails short and neat and apply a nail-sealing topcoat daily to strengthen the nails while they recover. Whatever you do, don't apply colored polish for several weeks—the pigmentation may stain the thin nail plates. With some attention and care, your natural nails should be back in shape in no time!

The basics: moisturizer, an orange stick, a disposable file, and a buffing block slice.

getting started at home

There isn't much that's more enjoyable to me than an hour spent lounging at home, taking care of my hands and feet. And no wonder—an at-home manicure and pedicure combines relaxation, indulgence, and the pursuit of beauty . . . plus, you get a real sense of accomplishment once you're finished, and can admire your perfect digits and glossy nails.

For most women, their own home was the setting for their very first encounter with nail polish: A little girl would watch her mother, and soon enough there would be tiny spots of color dabbed on the ends of her own fingers. As she grew up, an at-home manicure could mark almost any occasion: a special date, a slumber party with friends, or just a sunny Sunday afternoon.

It's time to reclaim the at-home manicure! You can groom your hands, perfect your cuticles, and paint your nails in less time than it takes to go to a salon, with results that look as polished.

And indulgence? When you do it yourself, you're in control—essential oils, your favorite music, total privacy. It's all in your hands—literally—when you bring the polish to your bathroom (or bedroom, kitchen table, or back porch).

There's barely a thing that's done in a salon that you can't do yourself at home—better, faster, and for a lower cost. So what are you waiting for?

the instant medicine-cabinet manicure

Whenever I talk to my clients about taking care of their hands and feet at home, the conversation inevitably turns to one thing: brands. *Which lotion should I use on my legs? Whose cream should I use for my rough heels? What emollient will get my hands perfectly soft?*

The answer is simple: Brand doesn't matter! There are no magic potions out there, made from rare flowers and bottled by monks at every full moon, that will miraculously change your life.

There are no **magic potions** out there.

More important than the brand, or even the ingredients list, is one simple question: *Will you use it every day?* The single most important element of nail care—in fact, of any element of personal care—is commitment to your regimen.

Still, we all are a little bit of a product junkie. I know I am, and will always be one. There. I said it. You're not alone. Your concoction of choice may be a drugstore brand with bright packaging and a range of complementary products, or the limited-edition boutique formulas that contain exotic ingredients and cost the same as a gourmet dinner for two. Either way, odds are good you've got a drawer (or a box, medicine cabinet, or even a closet) full of half-used tubs and tubes that . . . well, that seemed like a good idea at the time.

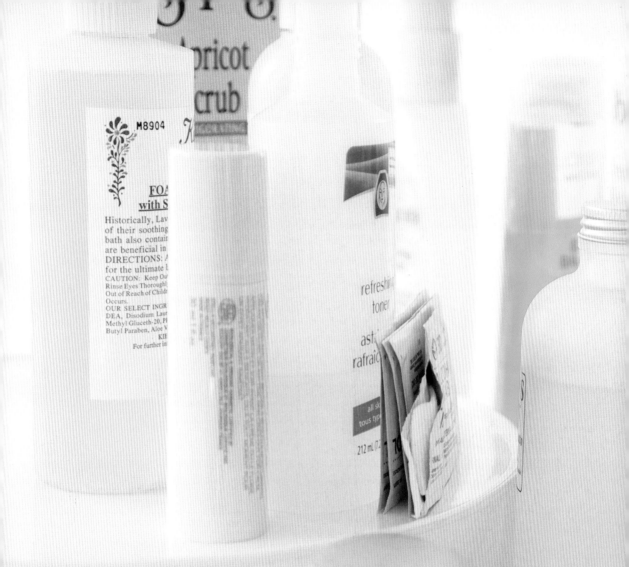

Virtually any beauty product can be repurposed for use on your hands and feet.

daily medicine-cabinet hand regimen

Before bedtime, use a facial scrub to exfoliate your hands, and rinse it off. Apply eye cream or antiaging serum to your cuticles and push them back gently, using your fingertips. Clean off excess oil or serum from your skin using a soft towel or tissue, and daub an antiaging product (one with AHA or glycolic acid) onto any sunspots or age spots. Slather your hands with night cream or eye cream, rub it in, and have a great night's sleep! If you're worried about getting the products on your sheets (some antiaging ingredients can discolor fabric), pull on a pair of cotton gloves before tucking yourself in.

Breathe easy—this beautifier reject drawer is a blessing in disguise! Virtually every product for face or body can be repurposed for use in hand and foot care—you probably have everything you need for an überluxe manicure right in your own medicine cabinet.

■ **Dump and organize.** It's time to take a deep breath and face your beautifier rejects. Dump everything out—everything—and organize all the items by expiration date. Toss *everything* that's past its prime, no matter how expensive it was or how good it still smells.

■ **Inventory.** Looking at your culled collection, take note of what you've already got. Break down your products by anatomy: face (cleanser, scrub, toner, moisturizer, special formulas for eyes) and body (cleanser, scrub, oils, creams, and lotions). Any prescription creams or serums shouldn't be included—use those only as your doctor recommends.

■ **Patch test.** Because you're now using your products for a more creative use than they were originally meant for, be sure to do a quick patch test on your inner wrist: Apply a dab of product and rub it in. If any reaction appears (sometimes it can take up to 24 hours), throw the product away. If your reaction is severe, call your doctor for advice.

Everything you've kept should fit into one of the categories listed in the next section. Even if you found that a product wasn't quite right for its intended use, it could be just the thing you need for your at-home manicure.

lotions & potions

facial products

When it comes to repurposing beauty products, there's an easy rule of thumb: *If it works for your face, it works for your hands.* The skin on your hands is a bit hardier than that on your face, but the chemicals and emollients in facial cleansers, moisturizers, and serums can work their magic anywhere on the body.

■ Facial scrub

If you've got a facial scrub that you don't use, take this miracle product out of the reject pile and put a container of it next to both your bathroom and kitchen sinks. This is a great way to incorporate exfoliation into your hand care regimen. 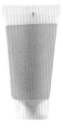 Designed to be gentle for delicate facial skin, these products will slough off the dead skin that creates rough patches on your palms and fingers.

■ Facial moisturizer

As gentle as facial cleanser, facial moisturizer is the ideal hand lotion—and if it has SPF, that's even better! If the bottle is portable, carry it with you in your makeup

■ Facial cleanser

Most face cleansers are ultragentle formulas, and they're perfect for mixing with warm water for soaking your cuticles. Cleanser's less abrasive formula helps keep your cuticles—which are prone to drying out—moisturized and soft.

pouch or handbag, and apply the moisturizer to your hands regularly: while you're at work, out for the evening, and especially traveling (dry airplane air is a death sentence for the delicate skin on your hands).

■ Toner

Toners that contain alcohol will strip your hands of their moisture barrier, drying out your skin. These shouldn't be used, but any toners that are alcohol-free can be swabbed onto the backs of hands and fingers with a cotton ball for a quick cleansing before moisturizing.

■ Eye cream

Most eye creams on the market are rich with vitamins and intense moisturizers, making them absolutely perfect for your cuticles and the back of your hands. Plus, eye creams often have lifting or antiwrinkle formulas that can help offset visible signs of aging, such as spots and thin skin. Apply these rich creams every night just before you go to bed, so your skin can absorb their dense concentration of nutrients and hydrators during the night.

■ Antiaging, alpha hydroxy, and glycolic acid products

Many people excitedly buy antiaging products, only to discover that their acidic formula is too harsh for the delicate skin on their face. But what's too much for your cheeks is exactly right for your hands, where the skin is hardier and the signs of aging are less insidious. Some of us have hardening cuticles or calluses forming around the edges of our fingers, and the mild acids in antiaging products help break

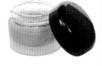

down the buildup of this rough skin. Antiaging formulas also serve as a terrific treatment for sun-damaged skin or age spots. Just dab it on before you head for bed. (But be sure to test it on a small patch of skin first—these products can be harsh.)

■ Night cream

Say it with me now: What's good for your face is *great* for your hands! The nutrient-rich formulas of most facial

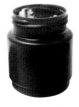

night creams are perfectly beneficial for the hands, too. Like eye creams, night creams should be applied to the hands just before going to bed, so that they have hours and hours to work their magic.

■ Body cleanser

Usually a little stronger and more heavily scented than facial cleanser, body cleanser nonetheless often contains moisturizing elements such as vitamin E or shea butter.

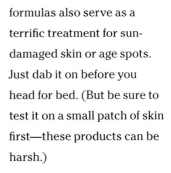

body products

In general, body products are less delicate than products designed for the sensitive skin of the face.

Use a drop or two in warm soapy water for soaking your cuticles, or even as a hand wash to keep at the sink.

■ Body moisturizer

Lotions, creams, and other moisturizers all transition seamlessly to a new life as hand cream. Keep large pump-top bottles or big tubs of cream near your bed, the bathtub, and the kitchen sink. Apply the lotion to your hands whenever you wash, whenever you change the channel, whenever you're bored . . . whenever!

■ Body exfoliant

A little rougher than facial exfoliants, body exfoliants are great for attacking trouble patches on the hands. They're also *great* as exfoliants for the tough, dry skin that tends to build up on the soles of your feet and the backs of your heels. Scrub your feet every day in the shower and you'll start noticing a difference almost immediately.

■ Body oil and bath oil

Anything with "oil" in its name is going to be a blessing for your cuticles. The intense, concentrated moisturizing properties of these oils will be evident with just a few drops applied to your fingers and toes, after bathing or before going to bed. Once you've oiled your cuticles, you can lotion up the rest of your hands and feet with a regular moisturizer.

do-it-yourself exfoliators

If you don't unearth any facial or body exfoliators while you're going through your beautifier reject drawer (see page 20), don't rush out and buy any! You can make phenomenal all-purpose scrubs with ingredients found in your kitchen or pantry.

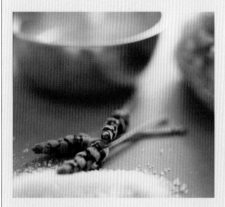

SIMPLE SUGAR EXFOLIATOR

This sweet treat sloughs off dead skin without being too abrasive. Just combine two parts granulated sugar (not powdered or superfine—the grains are too small) to one part body lotion, cream, or oil. Mix them together until you have a thick paste, scrub your hands and feet with it, and rinse thoroughly. Store any excess in an airtight jar labeled with the date—it will keep for up to a week.

If you don't even want to leave the kitchen, olive oil is an amazing base, and a little zested lemon peel helps mask the scent. If you use a nut oil—walnut, almond, or peanut—add a few drops of vanilla along with the sugar for an amazing dessert-scented scrub. And a pinch of herbes de provence *(or the contents of a tea bag in your favorite flavor) can turn a scrub based on corn or canola oil into a soothing aromatherapy experience.*

TROPICAL FRUIT EXFOLIATOR

If you want to go completely natural, turn to the produce section: Pineapple and papaya are both rich sources of alpha hydroxy acid (AHA), a powerful natural exfoliant. Just be sure to rinse off well so the natural sugars don't leave your limbs sticky.

Whichever fruit you use, start with a ripe, good whole one. Peel it and cut off the flesh (set it aside for a smoothie or fruit salad!). What you're looking for is at the center: The core of a pineapple or the pit of a papaya (with a bit of the fruit still clinging to it) makes a wonderful hand-held buffer. Roll it in sugar and gently scrub your arms and legs, paying special attention to rough spots and calluses. If the sugar dissolves, simply recoat the core or pit and dive back in.

For a bit of a boost, add a pinch of finely ground coffee to your sugar: The caffeine has been shown in some studies to boost circulation—plus, it smells heavenly with the sweet fruits!

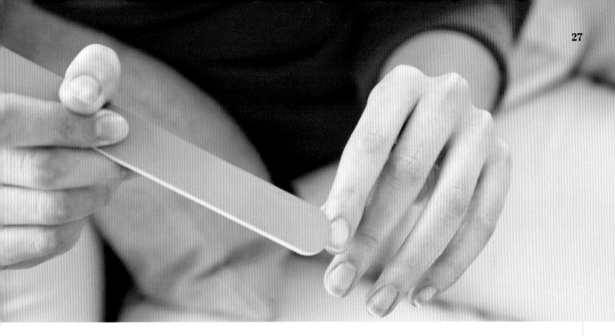

tools of the trade

AN ILLUSTRATED GUIDE

"Where did you buy your tools?" is the first question I ask a client who brings in her own manicure kit. I find it a continuing source of wonder that she usually can't remember where or when. Not even the slightest clue. Some manicure kits came as a free gift with a purchase at a long-forgotten makeup counter, some are passed down from mother to daughter like a family heirloom, some are left by visiting relatives or friends, some are swiped from hotel rooms, and some—a blessed few!—are actually bought with the intention of using them for nail care. Wherever they actually came from, odds are good they haven't been used in so long that they might as well have been unearthed from the attic.

If you've got your own tools, take a look at them. Are any of them nonmetal? Throw them out. In the trash. Forever. Plastic

The three varieties of nail file: metal, glass, and disposable.

rescue beauty lounge

tools can't be sterilized, and the risk of your plastic buffer or file containing oodles of bacteria is much too great for comfort. And take a good hard look at your metal tools before you decide that they're worth using again. Sure, it's less likely that you'll get a fungal or bacterial infection at home than you will at a salon, but it's still a possibility. Your tools always, always, *always* need to be sterilized.

Get a fresh start when it comes to your nail care tools. You don't need every tool on the list that follows, but make sure that you get the very best of whatever you do need.

Nail Files

Metal Files

There is a tremendous debate about whether metal files are healthy for your nails. In my opinion, metal files are the way to go! Not only can they be sterilized easily, but they also allow you to be more precise in your technique, creating smoother edges and more-even tips.

Glass Files

Fairly new to the market, the poreless surface of glass nail files makes sterilization a breeze. However, their dull grain makes it hard to file away a great deal of length. Reserve glass files for finishing touches, when their lightness and versatility truly have the chance to shine.

Disposable Files

While they're cheap per unit, disposable files (often called emery boards) turn out to be a big investment, since you *must* discard them after each use. Disposable files are measured in grades: The higher the grade, the finer the file and the softer and gentler it is. So if you have weak nails or have sensitivity when filing your

sharing tools

No one wants an infection. No matter how much you love your husband, or how much your sister's hangnail is annoying her, it's not worth using your own tools to help out. You just spread the risk of a bacterial or fungal infection.

Imagine this: A family member borrows your nail clipper and uses it to trim his toenails, and then he puts the clipper back where he found it without mentioning it to you. The next day, you take the clipper and trim your fingernails. Oh, and you have a habit of putting your finger in your mouth. And, oh dear, he might turn out to have athlete's foot, or a minor bacterial infection. And now it's been transferred to you.

Sure, this is an extreme case, but it's not all that hard to imagine. The time it takes to sterilize your tools before use, or even just to say no to someone who asks to borrow them, is nothing compared to the inconvenience and ick factor of realizing you've got an infection.

nails, choose the highest grade; if you have normal to thick nails, get a middle grade. Whatever grade you choose, though, buy in bulk, and look for the best price you can get. There are three types of disposable file, each with its own particular function. Here are the best of each:

Emery boards: inexpensive and available in a range of grades.

- **Fine grade:** Best for weak, brittle nails, the multidirectional grain sands your nail away gently and easily.
- **Medium grade:** Good for all nail types, its large end files your nails in one direction, while the narrow tip can be used for precision work, as well as to clean out under your nails.
- **Rough grade:** A rough, dense file for thick, stubborn toenails and heavy thumb edges.

Nail Clippers

Like nail files, different-size nail clippers are best for different uses.

- **Small:** Best for use on your fingers, and for anyone with tiny toes or weak toenails. If you have small hands, you might find these easier to use than larger clippers.
- **Medium:** Good for both hands and feet, and for weak to normal nails, this is the standard clipper that you'll find in most stores.
- **Large:** Ideal for thick, strong nails on big toes, for instance. This clipper shouldn't be used on weak nails, as it's likely to split the nail.

Nail Scissors

Nail scissors should be used only to trim the tips and corners of the nail—it's difficult to use them to cut off a great length of nail. Be sure the blades are sharp and straight, and be as attentive to sterilization as you would be with any other metal tool. If they become dull, they can be professionally sharpened.

Cuticle Pusher

Metal

As with metal nail files, metal cuticle pushers have some very vocal critics. They argue that this is a harsh method for pushing back your cuticles, since the metal can damage the nail root if you push too hard. I think that, whether it's metal or wood or plastic, *anything* can be dangerous and damaging if you use it incorrectly. The ease with which metal cuticle pushers can be sterilized makes them an invaluable tool in my book, and I strongly advise investing in one—or even two.

From top:
medium clipper,
nail scissors,
a metal cuticle pusher.

Cuticle pushers come in multiple shapes:

- ■ Generic: Good for all nail types, these have a straight end edge and a rounded end edge. Use the rounded end edge only—the straight one carries a risk of tearing your nail bed.
- ■ Rescue Beauty Lounge: The multifunctional, beveled edge metal makes it less likely that you will break your cuticles or push too deep.

Plastic

These are useful for getting past airport security, but not much else. Since they're not as sturdy as metal, I find that they bend too easily and are often too short for me to get a good grip.

Wooden Orange Stick

The classic multifunctional nail care tool, I adore these for almost everything, and use them all the time. But take note—orange sticks have to be discarded after each manicure, so it makes sense to buy them in bulk, cut them in half, and store them in an airtight container or Ziploc bag.

Wooden orange sticks

Cuticle Nippers

Nippers are quite technically challenging to use, especially on yourself! It requires skill and practice to trim evenly around your cuticles, and the potential for injury is high—especially if you're using your nondominant hand. I do not recommend using this tool at home, but if you must, use with caution—practice makes perfect.

Cuticle nipper

Cuticle Scissors

Instead of using the nipper (practise required!), use these specially curved scissors. They're great for trimming hangnails—especially if you're not technically precise or you're using your nondominant hand.

From top to bottom:
buffing blocks, a nail brush,
a pumice stone.

Buffing Block and Disk

A buffing block or disk is a must-have item—it primes the canvas for applying nail polish. The best buffers available are the disposable kind, and they aren't expensive. As with all disposable nail tools, you'll have to use a new one with each manicure. You won't wear down an entire buffer with one use, so you may want to make a batch last longer: Simply cut a rectangular buffing block into four parts. I like to buy buffers in bulk, cut them all up at once, and store the pieces in an airtight container or Ziploc bag.

Nail Brush

This is a must if you garden, cook, paint, or do anything else that gets the tips of your nails dirty. Since most nail brushes are made of plastic, it can be tricky to get them totally germ-free. This is not a disposable item per se, but you can only stretch its life out for so long—don't be afraid to toss yours every few months and buy a new one. If you're a nail brush devotee, you might consider keeping dedicated nail brushes in specific places: the kitchen, the bathroom, the garden sink, etc.

Pumice Stones

I'm probably going to get strung up for saying this, but here it is: I am not a fan of pumice stones. They slide around on the sole of your foot without actually doing any exfoliating, they're damp, warm havens for bacteria, they leave a grimy footprint wherever you let them rest, and they're impossible to sterilize. Get a rasp or a foot file instead.

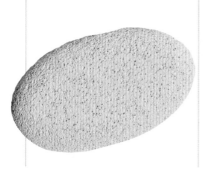

Foot File

There are several types of foot files, and like nail files, they vary in terms of both grade and durability. While disposable files are inexpensive, you pretty much have to buy a new one for each use—which, costwise, can add up. Considering the quality and long life of metal, with proper care they can more than pay off the initial investment.

- **Plastic:** These sheets of sandpaper glued to a plastic paddle work great the first time, but they go dull quickly. Even if the sandpaper file is advertised as reusable, don't. Reach for a new one each time—they work miracles.
- **Metal:** These hard-core metal files are meant for *serious* exfoliation, and do an amazing job with only a little bit of work. They're easy to sterilize, but can go dull after many uses. Still, springing for a new file every year isn't such a bad investment if it becomes dull.
- **Diamancel:** This particular brand of foot file is coated in real diamond dust. Not only does it exfoliate like a dream, but it self-sharpens and is good—with regular sterilization— pretty much forever. It's of a fine grade, and so is best used for buffing after an intense exfoliation with a rougher file.

Ingrown Side File

This is a great gadget to have for those folks who have intense dead skin buildup around their nails, and need to break up the cuticles clinging around the nail like ivy. It's easy to use, and hard-to-reach corners are no match for its intelligently designed shape.

From left: a plastic foot file, a metal foot file, and an ingrown side file.

Spoon Curette

Similar to the side file, but with a tiny spoon-shaped tip, this is perfect for the ingrown-toenail sufferers who need to pay extra attention to dead skin buildup between the nail and the cuticle.

Foot Bath

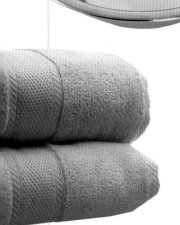

For soaking your feet during a pedicure, a bowl or basin is especially useful if you've mixed up a special soak that you don't want to get all over your bathtub. Plus, if they're metal, they're easy to sterilize in a dishwasher run on the "hot" setting.

Manicure Bowls

For soaking your fingers and mixing up scrubs.

Towels

For cleaning up spills, protecting tabletops, resting your wrists, and just general usefulness.

Cotton Pads and Swabs

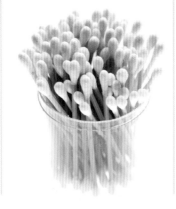

For polish removal, polish touch-ups, and cleaning off your tools. I don't recommend using cotton balls, as their fuzz tends to adhere to your nails, marring an otherwise perfect polish job. Instead, stick to square cotton pads and cotton swabs with the excess cotton twisted off. If you can find the swabs that have pointed tips, even better! They're perfect for precise touch-ups.

shopping list

For Hands

Nail clipper or scissors

Nail files of varying grades

Cuticle pusher

Cuticle-trimming scissors

Buffing block or disk

Nail brush (optional)

For Feet

Nail clipper or scissors

Nail files of varying grades

Cuticle pusher

Cuticle-trimming scissors

Foot files of varying grades

Buffing block or disk

Nail brush (optional)

General

Cotton pads

Cotton swabs

Ziploc bags

Lotions and Potions

Nail polish remover

Moisturizer

Exfoliators (fine for hands, rough for feet)

Cuticle oil

share love, not tools! make two separate kits . . . one for hands and one for feet

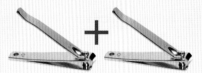

THREE WAYS TO
sterilize your tools

The truth is out there, and it's scary: Bacteria, viruses, and funguses all thrive where we tend to keep our personal grooming tools. Even if you thoroughly wash your implements after each use, there's still probably a swarm of nasty little guys that have taken up residence on your tools.

The answer, of course, is sterilization: killing all the germs. And fortunately for anyone who wants to avoid an infection, it's easy as pie. Whether it's for an at-home manicure or before bringing your own tools to the spa, you can effectively sterilize right in your own kitchen.

There are three basic methods of at-home sterilization: dry-heating, boiling, and soaking, and all take a lightning-fast 25 minutes (or less!). Make sure in any case that you are only sterilizing metal implements. Do not attempt to sterilize plastic or nonmetal tools.

Dry-Heating

Mise en Place

Mild detergent (such as liquid
   dish soap)
Metal tools to be sterilized
Cookie sheet
Solid metal tongs
   (no plastic grips)
Oven mitt
Ziploc bag

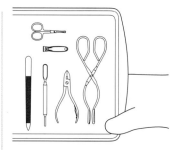

1. Preheat your standard gas or electric oven to 375°F.

2. Using hot water and mild detergent, thoroughly clean the nail implements, cookie sheet, and metal tongs to remove all visible debris.

3. Place the cleaned tools and the metal tongs on the cookie sheet, making sure they don't touch one another, and place the cookie sheet in the oven. "Cook" the tools for 12 to 15 minutes.

4. Wearing a clean oven mitt, carefully remove the cookie sheet from the oven and let cool. Using the hot tongs, place the sterilized tools in a fresh Ziploc bag. Write the date of sterilization on the bag with a marker and store your sterilized tools until their next use.

Boiling

Mise en Place

Mild detergent (such as liquid
   dish soap)
Metal pot
Metal tongs
Metal tools to be sterilized
Paper towels
Ziploc bag

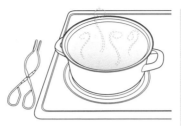

1. Fill the pot with water and place it on the stove over high heat. While you wait for the water to reach a rolling boil, clean your tongs and tools, using warm water and a mild detergent, to remove any visible debris.

2. When the water boils, use the tongs to place the tools in the boiling water. Don't drop them in—it will splash searing hot water. "Cook" the tools for 15 to 20 minutes, keeping the water at a rolling boil. Meanwhile, lay out several layers of clean paper towels and have a fresh Ziploc bag ready.

3. Dip the tip of the tongs into the boiling water for 60 seconds—this will kill surface bacteria on the tongs—and then use them to remove the tools from the water and place them on the paper towels.

4. Using the tongs, dry the implements on the paper towels. Don't use your hands! Not only are the tools (and tongs) very hot, but your hands will desterilize the surface of the tools, no matter how clean.

5. Holding the Ziploc bag open, use the tongs to place the dried tools inside. Seal the bag (you can use your hands now) and write the date of the sterilization on the bag. Store your sterilized tools until your next use!

Rubbing Alcohol

No kitchen? No oven? You can sterilize your metal tools by soaking them in rubbing alcohol (isopropyl alcohol) for 25 minutes. Put your tools in a pot, bowl, or even an upright glass and pour in alcohol to cover. When the 25 minutes are up, remove the tools, dry them, and store them immediately in a Ziploc bag marked with the date.

   Sanitizing your tools—giving them a quick swab-down with rubbing alcohol—is a superfast way to get rid of surface dirt, but not bacteria, viruses, and funguses. While it's better than nothing, it's not a true sterilization method.

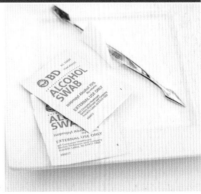

There's no place like home to make your nails look beautiful.

the at-home rescue manicure

Thirty minutes. Once a week. That's it. That's all the investment you need to make to have beautiful, well-groomed hands all the time. And while all our lives are busy—we juggle family, work, friends, and the million little things we always mean to get to—setting aside some personal time to take care of your nails can be a wonderful break from the everyday.

Becuase that's what an at-home manicure is: personal time. It's a chance to recharge, relax, and meditate—simultaneously taking care of yourself and making yourself just that little bit more beautiful and confident. Even if you don't have time to go through the whole routine, just knowing that you have the ability to take the manicure out of the salon and into your home can be an act of empowerment.

For me, my manicure time is a treat. I'm rarely standing still long enough to take a full half-hour for myself, but when I do make the time, it's magical. Turning everything off— my cell phone, my iPhone, my *other* cell phone—and just devoting that time to myself is restorative. Sure, it's glamorous to feel catered to by having someone else do your nails. But the feelings of meditativeness and accomplishment that come from doing your own manicure are irreplaceable.

manicure mise en place

For the basic at-home manicure, have all your tools laid out before you start.
Don't forget to sterilize your tools ahead of time! (See page 36.)

Tools

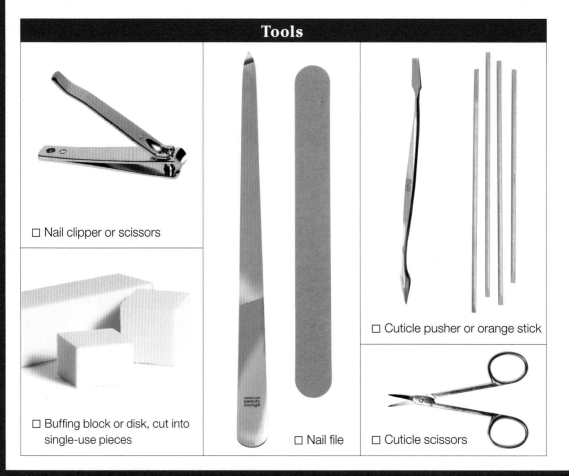

☐ Nail clipper or scissors

☐ Buffing block or disk, cut into single-use pieces

☐ Nail file

☐ Cuticle pusher or orange stick

☐ Cuticle scissors

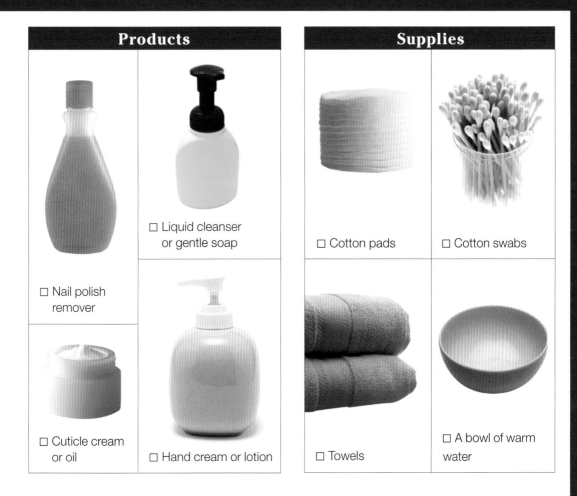

Products

☐ Nail polish remover

☐ Liquid cleanser or gentle soap

☐ Cuticle cream or oil

☐ Hand cream or lotion

Supplies

☐ Cotton pads

☐ Cotton swabs

☐ Towels

☐ A bowl of warm water

Getting Started

Once all your tools, lotions, and potions are ready to go, find a good place to sit. It should be somewhere with a comfortable seat—your favorite chair, your bed, even the floor with a cushion or soft rug beneath you—that is close to a flat, spill-proof surface on which you can set your supplies. I find it easiest to sit at a table with paper towels or an old cloth towel spread out in front of me.

Don't forget little touches—add candles, your favorite music, or a favorite movie playing in the background—which can help you feel more relaxed and help create a deep feeling of indulgence.

Start with a clean
slate: Remove your
polish completely.

STAGE ONE

trimming and smoothing

1 **If you're wearing nail polish,** remove it: Dip a cotton pad in nail polish remover and swipe it over your nails, pressing down firmly, until all the color is gone.

2 **Wash your hands thoroughly,** using warm water and soap, and dry them completely. If you have any residual moisture on your nails, the pressure of filing and buffing can cause weak nails to tear or split.

3 **Once your hands are bone dry,** take a good long look at your nails. Decide what length and shape you want them to be (see box, page 48). If you're not getting rid of very much length and need only to file your nails, skip to step 4.

When cutting your nails, always go from one corner of the nail to the other, using small, even snips. Never start with a large cut in the center, which can cause your nails to crack or split. If you're using scissors, keep the blade aligned with the natural line of your nails. To use a nail clipper, open the clipper by twisting around the lever and flipping it over. Slide the lip of the clipper under one corner of the free edge of your nail, making sure you're securely under the nail and that the line of the clipper follows the line of your nail. Cut each nail to an approximately even length. Don't worry about making it perfect—filing will smooth it out. Discard all your nail clippings into a trash can or onto a paper towel to be discarded later.

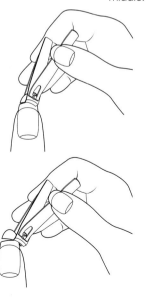

Always clip from one side to the other— never start in the middle!

Chapter Three

filing in the right direction

There's a debate that's been going on seemingly forever about whether it's okay to file in a back-and-forth motion, or whether you should only ever file in one direction. The answer? Both: If you have weak or fragile nails, file in one direction only, to avoid breakage. If your nails are healthy and strong, saw away! In either case, though, use long, slow strokes, not short choppy ones.

4 **Once your nails are the length you want,** it's time to file them into even shapes. If you're using a disposable file, strike the surface a few times with your buffer to dull it—it can be very sharp. But whatever type of file you're using, metal, disposable, or glass, the technique remains the same:

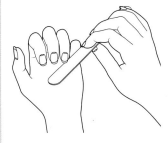

A. Rest the file between your thumb and your pointer finger, one-third of the way along its length, with your thumb pressed against the bottom side. Keep the rest of your fingers, except the pinky, on the top edge of the file. By freeing the pinky, you will have more flexibility and mobility when you file.

B. Keeping your hand relaxed, place the file between your nail bed and the underside of the free edge of your nail plate. Turn the file to a 45-degree angle, so that it is gently pressed against the tip of your nail.

C. Using long, even strokes, file your nail into an even shape. Don't use the short staccato motions that might be your habit—those can cause weak nails to split, and cause strong nails to become weak ones.

D. File each fingernail until they're all the same shape. Don't go too short, and don't file too far down into the corners of your cuticles.

A reusable metal file held at a 45° angle ensures a smooth finish.

A white buffing block cut into quarters is the perfect size for a single use.

5 Now that your nails are filed to an even length, it's time for buffing. Take your slices of buffing disk or pieces of block and, using the rougher side of your nail file, slightly dull the surface of the buffer (three to four strokes should do) to even out the buffing surface and protect yourself from any deep scratches.

A. Using the rough side of the buffing block, gently buff underneath the free edge of your nail. Smooth out all rough edges that might be left from filing.

B. With the pointed edge of the softer side of the block, delicately remove any debris that's trapped under the nail.

C. If you have deep ridges on the top of your nail, use a few strokes of the buffer to gently sand them down: Starting with the rough side, use an *X* motion—from the lower left of the nail to the upper right, and then from the lower right to the upper left. Follow that with a gentle side-to-side buff using the softer side of the buffer. Just a few seconds with each side should be enough.

D. If there are any lingering spots of roughness on the nail, use the softer side of the buffer to smooth them out.

6 Using an orange stick or cotton swab, remove all debris on the surface and underside of the nail.

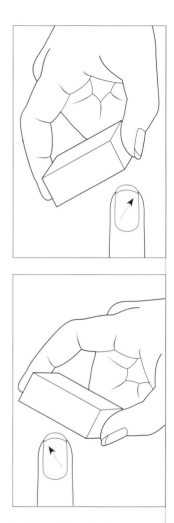

Buff in an *X* motion to smooth out ridges and imperfections.

shaping up

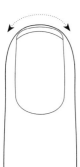

To achieve a short and natural shape, trim nails very short and file along the natural edge of the nail.

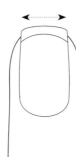

To achieve a square shape, trim straight across.

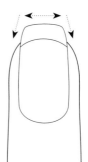

To achieve a square oval shape, trim straight across, then trim both corners at an angle.

short and natural

Are you the sort of person who thinks your nails are too short for a manicure? Short nails can be the epitome of chic, especially as a canvas for out-there colors. The key is to make sure the edges follow your natural shape—although everyone's free edge follows a different line, for most people it is a mirror of the shape of the fingertip. This low-maintenance look is perfect for those who work with their hands.

square

If you have weak nails that often break, or you just have small nail beds, this is the ideal shape for you. While the silhouette might be too angular on long nails, the straight, even surface can withstand the wear and tear of heavy daily use. Just be sure to keep them short so the edges don't chip off.

square oval

The "squoval" is the most popular nail shape in the business. Straight across the top and rounded at the edges, the square oval elongates the fingers and gives your hand a more feminine look. This shape is best if you have longer, stronger nails because filing the edges can cause weak or brittle nails to tear. And remember, the longer your nails, the more maintenance they'll require, particularly if they are in an angular shape like the squoval.

The shape of your nail is a matter both of aesthetics and of practicality. Along with color and length, the shape you choose for your fingernails can speak volumes about who you are and how you want the world to see you.

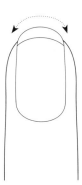

To achieve a round shape, don't cut straight across. Instead, follow the natural curve of your nail.

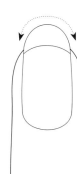

To achieve an oval shape, trim down one side, creating a curved edge, and then repeat on the other side.

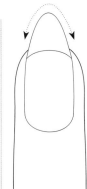

Follow the instructions for trimming the oval, but create a triangular point at the tip.

round

Because nails naturally grow in a somewhat rounded shape, this is a great silhouette for men and for those of us who need beautiful nails without a lot of hassle. Round nails look best short, making them ideal for people whose hands tend to get dirty (this means you, gardeners and cooking aficionados!). Also, if you've got wide nail beds, the all-around tapering will make them look slimmer.

oval

If you're lucky enough to have a job that doesn't require a lot of typing or general hand use, the classic oval is a beautiful, elongating look. Like a round nail, the oval is relatively natural looking, but it works best on a longer nail, because you'll need more space to form an oval shape. Wearers beware: This look works only if you are vigilant when it comes to filing, because typing, even on your phone keypad, will flatten an oval into a squoval in no time flat!

pointed

This nail shape is not for the faint of heart. But if you simply covet the lacquered talons of old-school Hollywood vixens like Bette Davis, then perhaps you've got what it takes. You'll need a few things in order to successfully pull it off: super-strong and long nails, a penchant for filing, lots of attitude, and a job that doesn't require (any) manual work. In fact, you may have to hire a staff to button your shirts!

STAGE TWO

cuticle care

cuticle pushing

Do it again! This is why I love doing manicures at home: You can push back your cuticles as many times as you like. Often at the salon, there's too much of a time constraint for your technician to be willing to put on more cuticle cream, let you soak your nails again, and push back your cuticles one more time. But there's no rule about how many times you get to push them back when you're at home—moisturize, soak, and push as much as you want. Plus, it's healthier than trimming—the more you push, the less you need to cut.

1 **Add some soap or facial cleanser** to your bowl of warm water. Add a few drops of cuticle oil if your cuticles are dry. (Avoid soap altogether if you have extremely dry cuticles.) Dip the fingers of one hand in the mixture to moisten them, and then generously apply cuticle cream or cuticle oil to the top of the nails. Rub it in gently and briefly.

2 **Soak your hand for a few minutes in the warm,** soapy water mixture. Luxuriate in the warmth, close your eyes and listen to music, or just let yourself drift off. Once your fingers are done soaking—how long that takes is your call, but I like to get my fingers out before the water starts getting cold—remove them and lightly towel off the excess moisture.

3 **Using the cuticle pusher or orange stick,** gently push your cuticle away from the nail. Be thorough: Get to all three sides of the nail (bottom, left, and right), as well as removing any dead skin that might have built up between the nail and the cuticle.

4 **Repeat steps 1 to 3** with the other hand.

5 **Massage another drop of lotion, cream, or oil** into both hands.

Just a few minutes a week with a cuticle pusher can keep your fingers gorgeous!

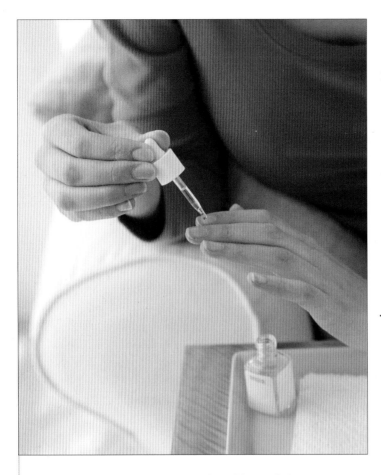

Cuticle oil provides
essential moisture.

6 **Using the buffing block or disk that** you used in stage one, do a final tidying-up inspection of the nails on both hands: Sand down the rough edges, evening out any asymmetries. Take an orange stick or the round end of your cuticle pusher and thoroughly clean out the underside of your nail using a side-to-side motion. Discard any debris.

7 **Do one final, gentle push back of your** cuticles using the orange stick or cuticle pusher (as in step 3 on page 50).

8 **Your hands should be completely dry by now.** If you like, without using soap, scrub down your nails with a dry nail brush to remove excess debris.

9 **Using your cuticle scissors, very carefully trim off the** dry skin or hangnails that were lifted when you pushed your cuticles back. Don't overtrim! We need our cuticles to protect the nail matrix from bacteria and other harmful elements. If your cuticles are in a state of crisis—they're very dry, or they've been cut (or bitten—oops!) to the quick—try not to cut them at all, unless it's an absolute emergency.

STAGE THREE

finishing up

1 Take a look at your nails. They should be beautifully shaped and even in length, with smooth, healthy-looking cuticles. If anything looks amiss, go back and fix it.

2 Using a nickel-size amount of exfoliating cream, scrub your hands and forearms gently for about sixty seconds. Don't rub too hard—the exfoliating agents can do their work with only a little pressure. Rinse or wipe off the exfoliator completely with a damp paper or cloth towel.

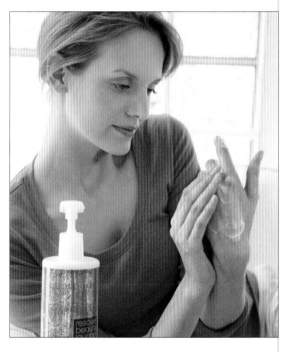

3 Moisturize! Using a lotion, cream, or other emollient, massage a generous portion into your hands and arms. Take your time—rub in gentle, firm strokes until the cream is completely absorbed. Pay special attention to your pressure points: the insides of your wrists, the heel of your thumb, and the spaces between your fingers.

Moisturizer helps lock in all the good work you've just done.

4 If you like, treat yourself to a damp towel warmed in the microwave for a few seconds (no more than 20). Wrap your freshly moisturized hands in the towel. Rest there for a minute, or until the towel cools. The warmth helps the moisture penetrate your skin—and, let's face it, it just feels amazing.

STAGE FOUR

cleanup

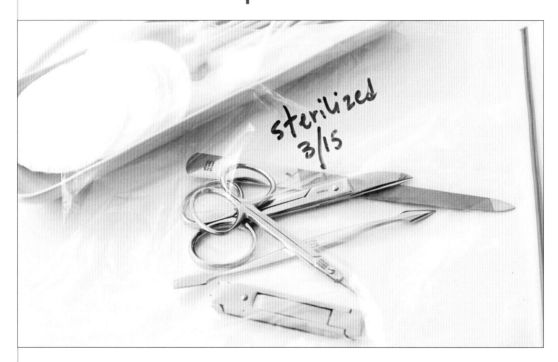

A dated Ziploc bag is the ideal storage for newly sterilized tools.

Once your hands are finished, it's time to make sure your surfaces and equipment are ready for your next manicure. Discard any trash, debris, and nonmetal implements. Scrub any metal or glass implements under hot water using antibacterial soap and a nail brush, and prepare them for sterilization (see page 36).

Admire your perfectly groomed hands! If you're planning to apply polish, see chapter 5 (page 72) for how to do it flawlessly.

manicure summary

mise en place

Set yourself up somewhere comfortable, with a flat work surface, and gather the tools and products listed on page 40.

trimming and smoothing

1. Remove old nail polish.

2. Using warm water and soap, wash your hands and dry them.

3. Cut or file your nails to your desired length.

4. File your nails into even shapes, using long, even strokes.

5. Using your buffing block, smooth out all rough edges that might be left from filing.

6. Remove all debris on the surface and underside of the nail using an orange stick or cotton swab, then wipe down using a damp cloth.

cuticle care

1. Add some soap or cleanser to your bowl of warm water. Moisten your fingers, and then

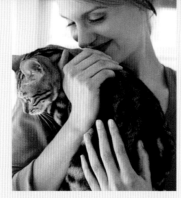

apply cuticle cream or oil to the tops of your nails.

2. Soak one hand for a few minutes in the warm soapy water mixture. Gently towel-dry.

3. Using the cuticle pusher or orange stick, lightly push your cuticle away from the nail.

4. Repeat steps 1 to 3 on the other hand.

5. Massage some lotion, cream, or oil into both hands.

6. Do a final tidying-up inspection of the nails, and buff or file wherever necessary.

7. Do one last, gentle push of your cuticles using the orange stick or cuticle pusher.

8. Completely dry your hands. If you like, scrub with a nail brush.

9. Use your cuticle scissors to very carefully trim off dead skin. Don't cut any live skin!

finishing up

1. Make sure your nails are even, smooth, and clean.

2. Scrub your hands and forearms with exfoliating cream for about 60 seconds, and then wipe it off using a damp towel.

3. Massage a generous amount of moisturizer into your hands and arms.

4. If you like, warm a damp towel in the microwave for a few seconds, and wrap your hands in the towel.

cleanup

Discard any trash, and store any glass or metal tools in a Ziploc bag until you're ready to sterilize them for your next use.

Admire your beautiful hands!

There's nothing
like perfectly
pedicured toes!

the at-home rescue pedicure

From teetering stilettos to summers full of endless flip-flops, we have a bad habit of sacrificing our feet for the sake of beauty and convenience. Just think how wonderful it feels to come home at the end of the day and slip off your shoes—now imagine creating that "ah" moment, without all the discomfort and pain that came before it! An at-home pedicure can work wonders.

O f course, it goes without saying that the hour (Really! Less than 10 minutes each day!) you spend giving yourself an at-home pedicure is also a great chance to relax, catch up with yourself, and spend some time just being away from the pressures of everyday life. Plus, you can sing along to your favorite music as loud as you want or catch up on your TiVo—which tends to be frowned upon in most nail spas.

Feet are pretty special parts of our body. We treat them to beautiful coverings: shoes that make our hearts skip and our eyes sparkle. But while the shoes are sleek, cool, architectural, brilliant—our feet within tell yet another story.

They're beaten up and abused to a staggering degree: carrying our weight all day, squashed most of the day in the moist darkness of a shoe, crammed into pointed toes, constricted by tight straps, and precariously balanced on spindly heels. And they show it.

pedicure
mise en place

Having all your tools and ingredients arranged ahead of time helps make the process of an at-home pedicure easier—you won't have to jump up and track wet footprints through the house trying to find your foot file! Be sure that your implements have been sterilized, see page 36 for instructions.

Tools

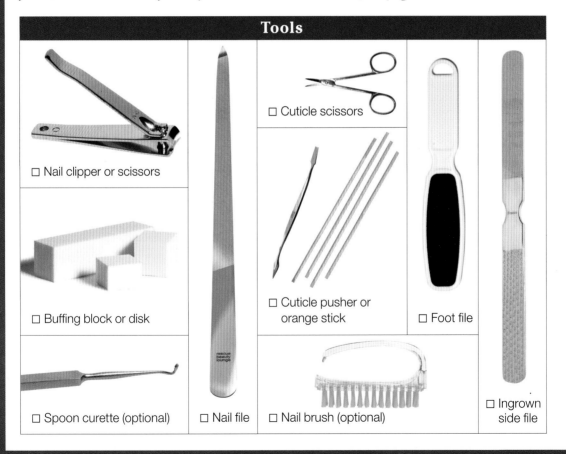

☐ Nail clipper or scissors

☐ Cuticle scissors

☐ Foot file

☐ Buffing block or disk

☐ Cuticle pusher or orange stick

☐ Spoon curette (optional)

☐ Nail file

☐ Nail brush (optional)

☐ Ingrown side file

Products

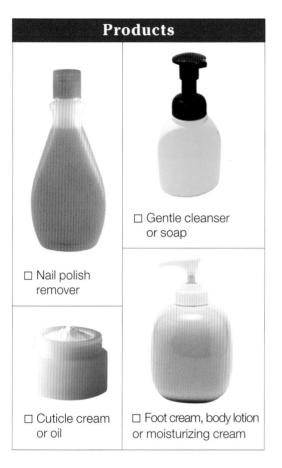

☐ Nail polish remover

☐ Gentle cleanser or soap

☐ Cuticle cream or oil

☐ Foot cream, body lotion or moisturizing cream

Supplies

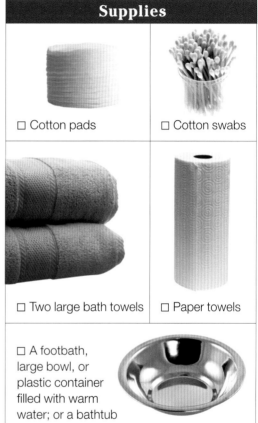

☐ Cotton pads

☐ Cotton swabs

☐ Two large bath towels

☐ Paper towels

☐ A footbath, large bowl, or plastic container filled with warm water; or a bathtub

LOCATION, LOCATION, LOCATION

When you've got everything ready to go, you'll want to find a good spot to give yourself a pedicure, a place where you can sit comfortably, as well as prop your feet up within easy reach. I find it

easiest to get set up in the bathroom, sitting on the lid of the toilet and resting my feet on the edge of the tub: I've got easy access to warm water, cleanup is easy, and towels are always at hand.

STAGE ONE:

getting ready

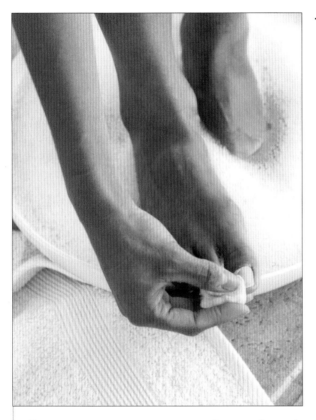

Be sure to remove
all old polish.

1 Set up shop at your workstation of
choice. If you're in a bathroom, fold
one of the large towels in half and drape
it over the edge of the tub where you'll
be placing your feet. If you're working
in another location, lay one of the large
towels on the floor where you'll be
working. Place your footbath or a large
bowl filled with warm water on the towel
and within easy reach. In front of the
footbath, fold the other towel in quarters
and place a sheet of paper towel on top—
this is where you'll rest your feet.

2 Remove old polish from your
toenails. Soak a cotton pad in nail
polish remover, and using firm pressure,
swipe the polish off each nail until it's
entirely clear of any residue. If you're
wearing a dark color, put a paper towel
under your feet—the pigments from the polish can seep into
cloth towels and ruin them.

Soaking your feet—here, an orange-mint
soak—is one of the best parts of stiletto rehab.

STAGE TWO

trimming and shaping

foot soaks

■ Heat 1 cup of milk in a microwave, and pour it into your soaking tub along with a few drops of your favorite essential oil. The lactic acid helps slough off your dead skin, while the oil provides soothing aromatherapy.

■ Add a few drops of oil to your favorite shower gel or hand soap, and add it to your soaking tub.

■ To create a luxurious, spalike atmosphere, float some flower petals, fresh herbs, or thin orange slices in your soaking bath. They may not do much therapeutically, but they look beautiful!

1 **Once your nails are free of polish,** it's time to trim them. If they are long, trim them using a toenail clipper or nail scissors. Cutting the nail on your big toe, which tends to be significantly thicker and larger than other toenails, is generally easier with a clipper than with scissors: Go from one corner of the nail to the other, using small, even clips. Don't do a big initial clip in the middle of the nail (that can cause pressure that can lead to cracking and splitting), and don't dig down into the corners of your toenails. For cutting the smaller nails on your other toes, either a clipper or a pair of nail scissors will do. Clip gently, and don't go too short! Discard all your nail clippings into a trash can or onto a paper towel to be discarded later.

2 **When your nails are the desired length,** shape them using a nail file. With filing, too, the big toe nail is generally better able to withstand pressure—and a rougher file—than are the more delicate nails on the other toes. (See the section on filing in The At-Home Rescue Manicure, page 44, for details on how to hold a nail file and where to place it against the nail.) On your other toenails, be sure to use a finer grade of file.

3 **After the nails are even in length and shape,** use your buffing block or disk to even out any visible ridges (which

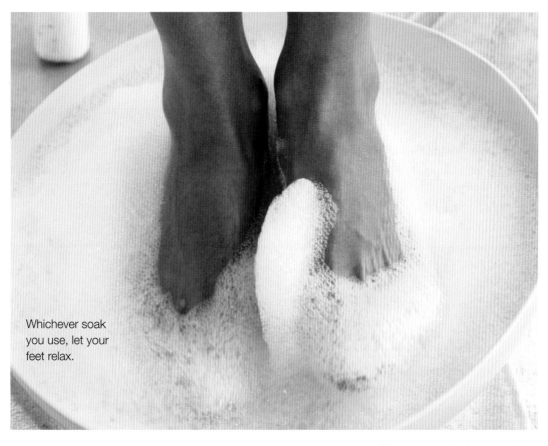

Whichever soak you use, let your feet relax.

generally appear on the big toe): Gently rub across the top of the nail with the rough side of the buffer, using an X-shaped stroke (lower left to upper right, lower right to upper left, see page 47). Using the softer side, buff in a side-to-side motion. Also using the softer side, gently buff across the top of the rest of your nails, just to smooth them out.

4 **Use an orange stick** or cotton swab to remove any debris from the surface and undersides of the nails. Discard the debris (onto a paper towel, if no trash bin is nearby), and moisten the tips of your toes with the warm water in the footbath or tub.

Clip your toenails from one side to the other—never from the center!

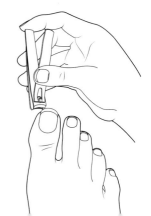

Tidy cuticles are a must for toes, too—apply cuticle oil liberally.

STAGE THREE

not-so-cuticles

1 Apply cuticle cream, moisturizer, or cuticle oil to the tops of your toenails and cuticles, rubbing it in gently but not all the way.

2 Put both feet—with the lotion or oil on your toes—into the footbath full of warm water. If you're working next to the bathtub, run the tub full of enough warm water to cover your feet, and dip your feet in. Sit back, soak, and relax. This is the best part!

3 Once you get fidgety (or the water gets cold—whichever comes first), take one foot out of the soak. Using a cuticle pusher or an orange stick, gently push back your cuticles. Make sure that you get the skin on all sides of the nail—left, right, and bottom—and that you pay special attention to the dead skin that tends to build up between the nail and the cuticle, especially on the big toe. If you have a spoon curette (see page 34), you can use it to really go at the dead skin buildup. Now do the other foot.

4 Repeat steps 1 to 3 on each foot: Apply lotion, soak both feet (add more hot water if necessary), and push the cuticles back on each toe. Repeat yet a third time, if you're so inclined.

special foot soaks

■ If you have discoloration on your toenails, try squeezing two lemons into warm water. Apply sage and lavender oils to the nails, and buff off the discolored surface with a buffing block.

■ Try soaking tired or achy feet in a warm footbath with half a cup of Epsom salts—it will remove odor and reduce swelling.

■ If your new summer sandals have left your feet blistered and swollen, take an ice water footbath, which will promote circulation, reduce swelling, and shrink blisters. An icy soak is also a perfect pick-me-up before a date or event.

STAGE FOUR

out, dead skin!

sandpaper foot files

I swear by sandpaper foot files. The body is plastic and looks like a paddle. It has two sides—rough/smooth. Start with the rough side, then finish up with the other.

The upside of the sandpaper file is that it's not expensive—you shouldn't pay more than $2 to $3 for one. The downside is that if you're giving yourself pedicures regularly, you're going to be shelling out for them every time: The sandpaper is usually of such a grade that it becomes dull after only one use. These can't be sterilized, and the paper becomes dull, so you should feel comfortable throwing them away after each use.

1 Now it's time for the fun part: exfoliation. Take one foot out of the water and gently towel it dry to remove any excess moisture. Your foot should be neither soaking wet nor bone dry, and still be soft from soaking. Holding your foot with one hand and your foot file with the other (this might involve pulling your foot up onto your lap), exfoliate along the rough edges of the sole using long side-to-side motions. Take your time and exfoliate well, dipping your file into the water every so often to keep it moist, and to rinse away the filings. You should see the dead skin come off—seriously! It's helpful to lay a few sheets of paper towel under your foot, to catch the so-gross-they're-almost-cool flakes of dry skin.

2 Keep exfoliating! Don't forget the sides of your feet, the tips of your toes, the inner corner of your big toe, the backs of your ankles, and—if you wear high heels a lot—the center of the ball of your foot. Stop exfoliating immediately if it begins to hurt or if your skin starts looking raw, but a little bit of redness is rarely anything to worry about. Once you've finished one foot, go on to the other. Do *not* resoak after you begin exfoliating. If your foot becomes too dry to continue effectively, moisten the file—not your foot—and keep exfoliating.

3 Discard all the accumulated dead skin and undesirable mess. Wipe your feet off with a fresh paper towel (a damp one is okay) to remove any debris that's left on the skin after exfoliating.

Exfoliating your feet—here, with a Diamancel file—is the best route to smooth heels.

You can never use too much
moisturizer. Be sure to get all
the way up your legs

STAGE FIVE

finishing touches

1 Take another look at your cuticles. If they need more attention—they might have crept back while you were busy exfoliating—moisten your toes and go back in there.

2 Using your cuticle scissors, trim the pushed-back skin and any hangnails that are on your toes. Don't clip too deep—a bloody mess doesn't make for a cute pedicure.

3 Go back over the tops and tips of your toenails using the buffing block or disk. Using the soft side, lightly brush across the tops of your toes to seal the nail, and use the corner of the buffer to clear up any debris left over from trimming your cuticles. Discard any mess.

4 Fill your footbath or bathtub with fresh warm water, and scrub your feet and lower legs with an exfoliating scrub using your hands or a fresh towel. (See page 26 for recipes on how to make exfoliants at home.) Wipe your legs clean with a towel, and gently pat them dry.

5 Rub a generous portion of moisturizer into your feet and legs. Press firmly and use long, vertical strokes, in order to best promote good circulation (plus, it just feels good!).

first aid

Accidents do happen—at home or in a professional setting—and most of the time they're due to overzealous cuticle cutting. Using only sterilized tools can give you peace of mind, but you should always stop immediately to take care of your injury. Disinfect the cut using antibacterial ointment, and bandage your finger or toe. Keep it protected until it's healed— there's no such thing as a germ-free environment.

STAGE SIX

cleanup

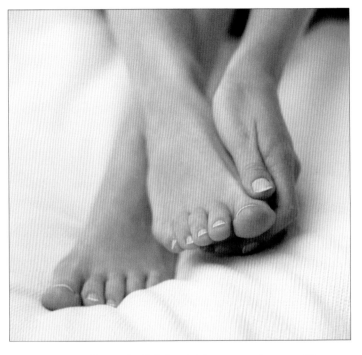

Perfection! Trimmed, filed, and buffed to their most beautiful state.

Once your pedicure is finished, it's time to clean up. Throw away any trash, debris, or nonmetal implements. Thoroughly clean any metal or glass tools with hot water and antibacterial soap, scrubbing them with a nail brush. Let the tools dry until they're free of moisture, and sterilize them for your next use (see page 36 for the sterilization how-to).

If you're going to polish your toes, check out page 80 for the instructions for a flawless finish. Polished or not, sit back and admire your pristine and perfect toes!

pedicure summary

mise en place

Sit somewhere comfortable where you can put your feet within easy reach. Gather the tools and products listed on pages 58–59.

getting ready

1. Set up your towel near a basin or bathtub, and lay out a paper towel for your feet.

2. Remove any old nail polish.

trimming and shaping

1. Trim your toenails to the desired length.

2. File your nails into even shapes, using regular strokes.

3. Using your buffing block or disk, smooth out any rough edges and the tops of the nails.

4. Use an orange stick or cotton swab to remove any debris.

not-so-cuticles

1. Apply cuticle cream or moisturizer to the tops of your nails and cuticles, and rub it in.

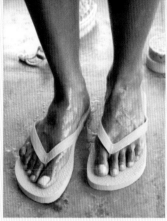

2. Soak both feet in your footbath or tub. Relax!

3. Take your feet out of the soak, and gently push back your cuticles using a cuticle pusher or orange stick. If you're using a spoon curette, remove any dead skin.

4. Repeat steps 1–3 on each foot—twice, if you like.

out, dead skin!

1. Use a foot file to scrub down all the rough parts of your foot, dipping the file in water occasionally to keep it moist.

2. Get at the hidden spots: the tips of your toes, the sides of your feet, the ball of your foot. Do *not* resoak your foot.

3. Discard any debris. Wipe your feet off to get those last bits of dead skin.

finishing touches

1. Reexamine your cuticles to see if they need more work.

2. Using your cuticle scissors, trim any pushed-back skin or hangnails.

3. Re-buff the tops and tips of your toenails, and use the corner of the buffer to remove any debris under the nail.

4. Refill your tub or footbath with warm water and, using an exfoliating scrub, slough your feet and up your legs. Wipe clean with a towel.

5. Rub moisturizer into your feet and legs, pressing firmly.

cleanup

Discard any trash, and wash off your glass and metal tools. Set them aside in a Ziploc bag for future sterilization.

Admire your beautiful feet!

All you need for a
perfect polish—right at
your fingertips.

polish perfection

What do most people picture when they think about manicures and pedicures? A set of shiny, flawless, glossy nails—in other words, the polish. But that's off the mark: The real *point* of the manicure or pedicure is the maintenance: soaking, scrubbing, trimming. *The polish is just the icing on the cake.* So many of my clients are slaves to their nail polish, terrified of their real nails being seen by the world. How silly is that? I say stop letting your polish control you—you control the polish!

For all that I insist the important part of the manicure is all that comes before the polish, I might as well face facts: The polish . . . well, it's the *popular* part. It's the pretty part. It's—okay, I'll admit it— the fun part. But, I do want to stress that nail polish or any other ornamentation is only that: ornamentation. Your nails should be in healthy, perfect condition whether they're polished or not, and you should never use polish to cover up unhealthy or poorly cared-for nails.

Still, I understand the obsession. I absolutely love nail polish: the glossiness of it, the way it makes nails look like glass or metal or as soft as a flower petal, the way you can express your inner fashionista, and, of course, the ease with which you can change from one color to another. At least it's easy if you know how to do it yourself. In this chapter, you'll see just how simple it can be—from sweet pinks to vampy black, your nails will be gorgeous!

nail polish application 101

oily nails

Just like our skin and hair, our nails can run the spectrum from dry to oily. There are some people who simply produce more natural oil than others, and nail polish has a hard time sticking to their nails.

To keep your polish adhered, you need to prep your nail plate. Before starting your manicure, scrub your nails with a clean nail brush and oil-free soap—dishwashing liquid, which is designed to cut grease, works wonders. Avoid any polish removers that have vitamin E or aloe—they will add oil.

The secret to a perfect nail polish application is simple. It's 50 percent preparation and 50 percent application.

Preparation? Yes, indeed. Just like refinishing furniture or painting the walls in your home, you need to have a clean, good work surface in order to get the best application of color. Regardless of the brand of polish you use, a smooth preparation will make the polish go on smoother, look prettier, and last longer. See page 39 for the At-Home Manicure, the perfect prep for perfect nails.

You can polish your nails almost anywhere, but be wary of wooden surfaces or painted furniture: The chemicals in the polish remover and the polish itself can strip the color or finish. If your only choice is a wood or painted surface, lay out some old cloth or paper towels.

Polish is best applied immediately after you've finished giving yourself a manicure (page 39) or pedicure (page 57). Your nails are clean, trimmed, and perfectly primed to receive color. Make sure that all the moisturizer you've applied is cleanly wiped off, though—an oily surface can make the color adhere unevenly, and may cause bubbling.

If you're planning to polish both fingers *and* toes, do your toes first (see page 78). That way your hands—unencumbered by a fresh coat of polish—can work freely.

mise en place

Supplies

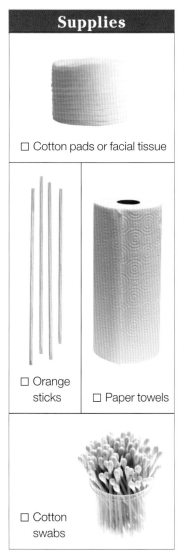

☐ Cotton pads or facial tissue

☐ Orange sticks

☐ Paper towels

☐ Cotton swabs

Products

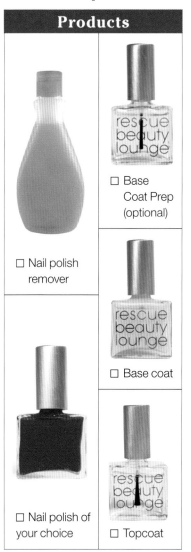

☐ Base Coat Prep (optional)

☐ Nail polish remover

☐ Base coat

☐ Nail polish of your choice

☐ Topcoat

base coat prep

Rescue Beauty Lounge was the first place you could get Base Coat Prep, and it was truly an idea whose time had come: It's a product we developed that helps your base coat stick to your nail—absolutely ensuring that there is zero oil or oil residue on the surface of your nails. It bonds the base coat on super tight, which helps the polish last practically forever. (Okay, 6 to 10 days.) Now a number of drugstore brands carry similar products—look for them under names such as "pre-base coat," or "base coat primer."

A matte nail is the ideal
platform for long-lasting
polish—base coat prep
helps you get there.

how to hold your hand

There are two dominant schools of thought as to how to hold your hand for self-polishing. The adherents of one like to have the hand laid out flat on a surface such as a table or countertop (lay down paper towels to protect the surface) and swipe the polish away from them. The others like to hold their hand in the air, palm toward them

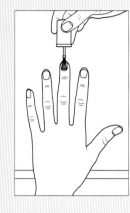

and fingers curled over, and swipe the polish toward them (or downward, depending on the angle of the wrist).

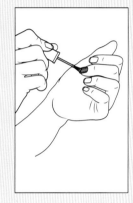

There's no right or wrong method. Do what works for you: what feels most comfortable, and what delivers the best results. You might find you even use one method for one hand and one for the other.

Polishing Fingers

Polishing fingernails is difficult, because the hand has to be both a canvas *and* a tool. Inevitably, you'll start out much better at polishing one hand than the other, but with practice and dedication you'll soon be able to crank out polish applications at home that rival any that you see done by a professional.

1 Your hands should be free of any nail polish before you start. If you've just finished giving yourself a manicure (see Chapter 3), you don't need to worry about removing polish, since you've already done it. But if you're jumping in here, soak a cotton pad in nail polish remover and firmly swipe away any polish or oil residue that's lingering on your fingernails.

base coat

Sometimes it feels as if there are a million versions of base coat on the market. Is there any difference among them? As it happens, yes. Try to find a base coat that advertises added vitamins or protein. It won't work miracles, but it helps keep your nails from becoming brittle, and bonds more strongly to your nails than the ones without do.

If you have irregularly colored nails, look for a base coat that's not entirely transparent. A milky sheen means that it will act as a color primer that mutes the natural color of your nail. This can help the color of the polish start with a blank canvas.

2 **Do it again.** No matter what state your nails are in—post-manicure, post-polish-removal, or totally virgin—clean the surface of your nails *again* with a cotton swab that's been dipped in nail polish remover. The chemicals in the remover lift off any oils that remain on your nails. They should look quite dull and dry. This is a good thing! It indicates that the surface is completely free of oil residue.

3 **If you're using Base Coat Prep,** apply it now to each finger, avoiding your cuticle areas. If you don't have Base Coat Prep, just move on to the next step.

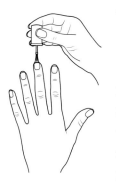

4 **Apply a thin layer of base coat** to each finger, one hand at a time, and let it *dry completely,* which can take up to 3–5 minutes. Seriously—let it dry all the way. This step is critical! Base coat is your foundation: It does double duty, protecting your nail plate from discoloration from the polish, and protecting your polish from the oils of your nail plate. Give it a chance to dry and adhere fully before going further.

5 **It's time to move on to color** once your base coat is dry. This requires practice, so be patient with yourself as you go—you'll become more comfortable and develop greater facility with time. For best results, I strongly recommend doing one hand at a time from here to the end: polish, topcoat, and drying time. Wait until one hand is completely dry before starting to polish the other one.

A. Set up your nail polish bottle so that it's in easy reach. If you place it too far away, the polish will start to dry on the brush in the few seconds it takes to move the brush from the bottle to your fingertip, and will become more difficult to manipulate.

B. As you remove the brush, bend it against the lip of the bottle to squeeze out excess color. There shouldn't be any visible drips, and the color definitely should not drip off the brush as it moves from the bottle to your hands.

C. Once you've brought the color to your fingers, fan the brush flat against the base of your pinky nail.

D. Using wide, even strokes from base to tip, *thinly* coat your nails with polish, moving from your pinky to the other fingers and ending with your thumb, one hand at a time. If you get some color on your cuticles, don't stress! You'll fix it later. Let the coat dry completely.

E. Once your first thin coat of polish has dried, go back for the second coat. (Unless you like the way only one coat looks—no reason to do two if you don't want to.) Repeat the process identically: a thin coat, even strokes, pinky to thumb. Work slowly, and don't be afraid of making mistakes—they're easy to fix!

6 When your color has dried completely, apply a layer of topcoat to each finger. Let it dry completely.

7 Dip the end of a cotton swab in nail polish remover and carefully get rid of any imperfections. Take care not to get remover on your perfectly polished nails!

8 Wait. Watch TV, listen to music, meditate . . . just don't *touch* anything until your nails are *completely* dry. Give yourself as much time as you can possibly stand—20 minutes would be ideal.

9 Admire your beautiful, shiny, glossy nail polish!

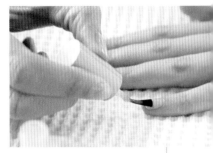

First base coat . . .

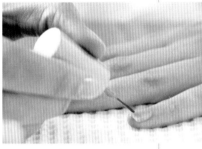

. . . then color . . .

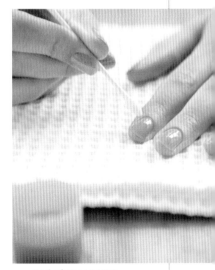

. . . and after topcoat, cleaning up the edges.

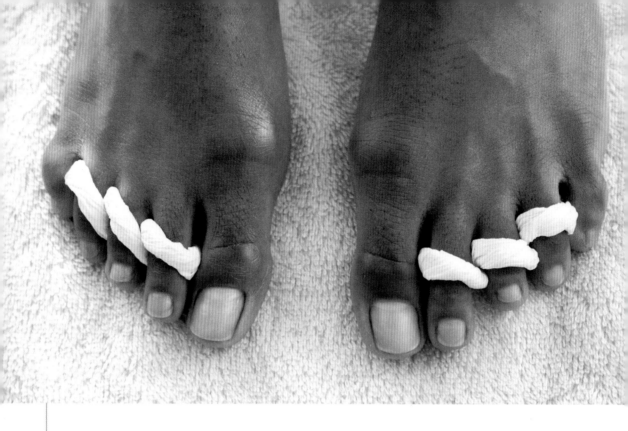

A toe separator made of paper towels is easy, hygienic, and inexpensive! Just twist the towel into a thin snake, and weave it through your toes—over, under, over, under—and back around. Tuck in the ends, and you're done!

Polishing Toes

Polishing your toes is pretty much identical to polishing your fingers, except a whole lot easier, since you've got both hands to control and coordinate your polishing. And you don't have to use one freshly polished foot as a tool to polish the other!

The big difference between polishing fingers and polishing toes is the necessity of keeping your toes separate, both so that they're easier to reach and so that they don't smudge each other like they would when they're in their natural state—most people's toes overlap slightly.

I'm not a fan of the foam toe separators that are sold at drugstores and come with pedicure kits—they're havens for germs and bacteria, and don't do anything that can't be done with a paper towel. Simply twist a sheet of paper towel into a thin snake,

chemicals and allergies

Nail polish is a complex cocktail of chemicals, and while it's harmless for most, there are some people who should be wary.

Many people have been concerned about allergies and ill effects as a result of toluene, formaldehyde, and DBP—chemicals that appear in some nail polish formulas. In response, a number of nail polish manufacturers have rushed to get to market new formulas that are free of these components. If it's something about which you're concerned, check the ingredients list before buying your polish—it's required that every ingredient be disclosed.

There have also been some recent studies that seem to indicate that nail polish can be harmful to women who are pregnant or nursing. For this—and any other serious concern—speak to your doctor. New studies are being done all the time, and a medical professional is the best authority.

Even if you find yourself unable to use polish, it's quite possible to have beautiful nails without it— just see the section on buffing on page 99.

and weave it between your toes. Tuck the loose end under a loop and poof! Instant toe separator!

People contort themselves into all sorts of positions to best reach their toenails. I've had great luck resting my feet against the ledge of a bathtub or the edge of a table. In that position, unlike bringing my foot up onto my lap, which is the other common method, there's no risk of smudging my polish against my arms or legs. But ultimately, what works best is whatever makes you the most comfortable and the happiest with your results.

Of course, you'll still want to control the amount of polish on the brush and paint on thin, even coats. But with toes, I find it easier to start with the big toe and move toward the pinky.

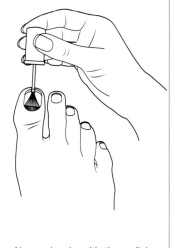

Always begin with the polish brush fanned at the base of your nail plate.

french manicure tips

Instead of a solid wash of color, the French manicure—sheer pink or white across all of the nail, with a strip of opaque white at the tip—can be a subtle and classic alternative. A few warnings: Your nail has to be slightly longer (but only a little: an eighth of an inch of tip is enough). Be wary of using a white that's too chalky, since white that bright will look too contrasting and unnatural.

Play around with your sheer and opaque colors until you find a combination that suits you. Instead of clear pink, try a clear beige or even a translucent white—the differences are subtle, but they speak volumes.

Here's my favorite formula for French manicures, which I especially love to see on brides.

1 Apply base coat prep and one coat of base coat as you normally would.

2 With a very sheer pink polish, apply two light coats, letting each dry thoroughly.

3 Using your soft, sheer white polish of choice, very carefully apply one or two thin coats to the very tip of the nail, following the nail shape.

4 If you want a more subtle look, top the entire nail with yet another thin coat of the sheer pink, let it dry, and then apply topcoat. Otherwise, go straight to the topcoat.

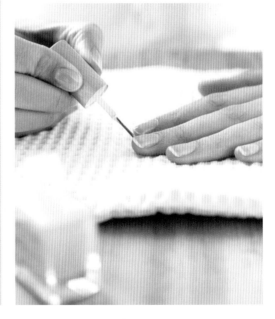

nail emergency 911

No matter how conscientious you are, it's inevitable: We all smudge! At home or at work, whether we did our own nails or had them done for us. Digging through your purse, typing on your cell phone, or opening the mail. You rap your nails against a sharp edge, or you just *have* to push your hair out of your eyes while your polish is drying, or some sort of inexplicable chemical reaction causes your polish to start bubbling up like a science-fair volcano.

If something happens to your polish—relax! no worries! Remember, it's easy to fix these little problems. It's just nail polish!

Bubbling Polish

When nail polish bubbles, it's for one of two reasons. First, because air has become trapped in the polish itself. This is an easy one to avoid: *Never shake a bottle of nail polish.* If your polish has become separated in the bottle, remix it by gently rolling it back and forth between the palms of your hands.

Roll—never shake—your polish.

The second culprit for bubbles in your polish is oil residue on the surface of the nail, which rejects the lacquer and pushes it away from the nail, creating a bubble. How do you get rid of this? When you're painting your nails in the first place, use nail polish remover—even on naked nails—to ensure that there's no oil or residue of any kind on the nail plate before the polish goes on. If this sort of bubble appears, your best hope is to take the polish off that finger and reapply it from the beginning, as outlined on page 77.

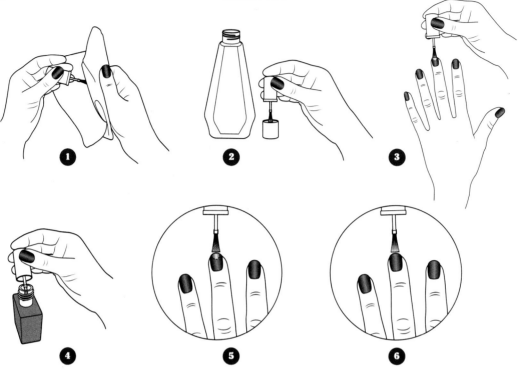

Chipped or Smudged Polish

Right off the bat, you need to determine if the chip can be filled in, or if you'll have to redo the entire nail. If you have a small chip on the tip that covers less than 20 percent of the nail plate, then you can proceed with an emergency fill. If it's a bigger chip than that, you're going to have to take the polish off and reapply, as explained on page 77. In either case, the most important thing is to have available the exact same nail polish color you're wearing.

To fill in a chip, get your nail polish remover, your nail polish, and your topcoat. **1.** Clean the brush of your nail polish with a paper towel that's been moistened with polish remover. (Be careful not to ruin your other, perfectly polished nails!) **2.** Dip the clean nail polish brush into some of the nail polish remover that's been poured into the cap.   **3.** Paint the nail polish remover onto your nail to even out the polish so that it's at the same level as the chip.   **4.** Once it's all even and has dried, clean the nail polish brush again with a paper towel, and this time dip it into the polish.   **5.** Using thin layers of color, fill in over the chip and any other part of the nail that needs another layer of color. Let it dry *completely*—at least 3 minutes, preferably 5—and apply another coat.   **6.** Once your second coat of color is dry, apply topcoat to the entire nail and let it dry completely.

Streaky Polish

Don't worry—it's not your fault if your nail polish is streakier than Cruella De Vil's hair! There are a few factors that cause polish to go on unevenly. Consider the polish: opaque whites and white-based pastels tend to streak because of the density of the pigment. Sheer, less densely pigmented colors go on smoothly. If you want to alter the intensity of the hue, apply several coats, but if you've got your heart set on a heavy polish, just practice on a sheet of paper before painting your nails. If it's not the polish, then the streaking is probably due to natural oil residue on your nail plate. After washing your hands with soap, swipe away the oil with nail polish remover and apply a Base Coat Prep (see page 75).

Bleeding Polish

It's really frustrating not to be able to take off all your nail polish when you want to, as many dark and pigment-rich colors will bleed into your cuticles and the skin around your nails. To get this color out, show no mercy! Really soak your cotton pad in polish remover, and be strategic in removal: Start from the cuticles at the base of your nail, and work toward the tip, angling the cotton pad away from your cuticles and in toward the center of the nail. And be generous with the remover!

There's a technique to get this color out:

Show no mercy!

the big spill

We've all done it: spilled bright red nail polish on a newly varnished table, dripped hot pink on white sheets, or knocked over a bottle of pearly white on a dark hardwood floor. Spillage is a risk we take for beautiful nails. There are only a few things you can do to remove pesky lacquer stains, and using nail polish remover is not one of them. Though it's great at removing color from nails and skin, it is formulated only for those uses.

If you do find yourself with an unwanted spot of polish on fabric or a hard surface, wait until the polish has dried. (You can try taking a few deep breaths and repeating the mantra "Out damned spot" à la Lady Macbeth if the spill's in a particularly inconvenient location.) If your drops are on a highly absorbent fabric such as cotton or silk, I recommend taking it to your dry cleaner right away—they see this sort of thing all the time. If the stain is on a smooth surface (a table or countertop, a hardwood floor), press a piece of Scotch tape over the dried polish, press it down, rubbing it in, and take it off in one quick motion. Continue taping and ripping until you've removed the whole spill.

If the spill is on a particularly prized surface, don't hesitate to throw up your hands and call a professional cleaner to do the dirty work for you.

Reviving Your Manicure . . . Quickly!

So you've got the perfect manicure. Whether you did it yourself or you had it done, you're happy and bubbly with your perfectly polished fingers. And then . . . *BOOM!* Just before that cocktail party, or a black-tie wedding, or an out-of-the-blue business meeting that can make or break your career, your once-perfect nails just don't live up to perfection. There might not be any chips or smudges, but the color looks dull and tired, and the shine isn't nearly as shiny as you'd like it to be.

If you don't have time for another full manicure, it's easy to revive a tired one. This is also great as a midweek, between-manicures pick-me-up! For a luxe touch, exfoliate your hands before getting started, and then wrap them in a warm, wet towel to rejuvenate your skin.

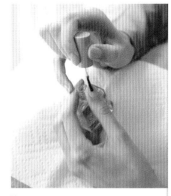

Topcoat . . .

1 **Wash your hands with mosturizer-free soap,** and dry your hands thoroughly.

2 **Apply topcoat to all your fingers,** and let it completely dry. If you're wearing dark polish, the topcoat will take longer to dry, so give yourself at least 15 minutes.

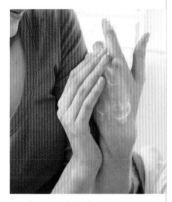

. . . then moisturizer . . .

3 **Once the topcoat is bone dry,** slather on hand cream or lotion. Let it soak in, and then rub the lotion residue off your nails.

4 **Give the tops of your nails** a quick shine using a snag-free cloth, such as microfiber or cotton (a T-shirt works perfectly), and go!

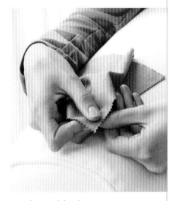

. . . then shine!

color theory

O h, the questions that color brings up. *What goes with this outfit? What enhances my skin tone? What should I wear to this particular event? What's trendy this season?*

They all have the same answer: Whatever you want. It would be great, wouldn't it, if I could give you a list of every color out there and tell you exactly when to wear it and precisely what it says about you. But the truth of the matter is that while yes, some colors might be a little bit more appropriate than others at certain times (wear acid green to a job interview at your own risk), the ease with which polish can be put on or taken off means that you can experiment—wildly and conservatively—and not feel the need to be a slave to standards or expectations.

There are a few bits of truth behind the myths, though: A pale, sheer white polish will beautifully offset tanned skin. Dark, lacquered red does send a seductive vibe. Classic pale pink can be worn anytime, anywhere. But the

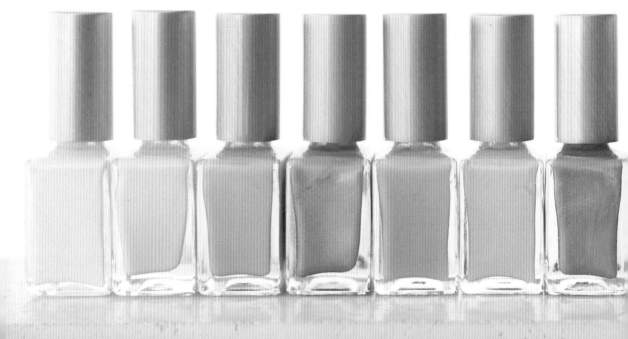

old rules about restricting more vibrant shades to your toes? Or wearing coral only if you're over 70 and out of touch with fashion? Or never wearing glitter if you're out of grade school? You can toss those out the window. The important thing is that you think your nails look beautiful. And if they're neat and well groomed, and your polish is applied evenly, your nails will look great no matter what color you choose to dress them in.

There are hundreds of nail polish brands out there, and they come in a zillion colors. When I opened Rescue, it didn't seem to me that the market needed a zillion and one. Still, the night before a fashion show one year, frantically mixing colors, we had an epiphany. I wanted to make a line of nail polishes that covered all the basics—and did it *perfectly.* And so our Rescue Beauty Lounge colors are what I think of as the perfect red, the perfect coral, the perfect metallic. The colors that follow are all Rescue Beauty Lounge brand, but they're reworkings of the classic hues, so slight variations on almost all of them can be found in any of the major nail care lines. And before you ask, no, I don't have a favorite. I love all these colors as if they were my children, and I wear them all.

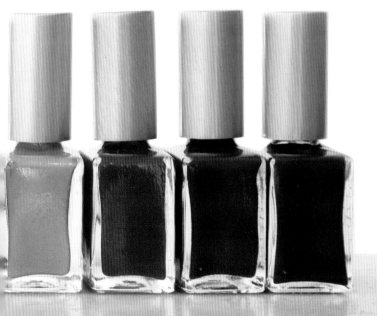

From sheer and pale to dark and sexy, the spectrum is yours to play with!

easy colors and hard colors

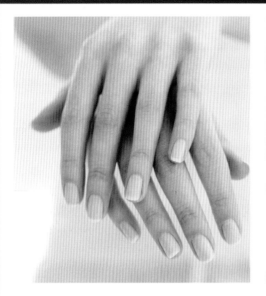

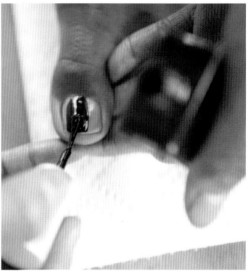

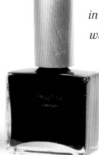

Clear Pink: easy

Not all nail polish colors are created equal. Very dark colors, pale colors with a white pigment base, and colors that are pearly or opalescent are just more difficult to apply than sheer, light polishes. It's partly a matter of any mistakes being more obvious, and it's also that the chemical makeup of the polishes makes these colors thicker and less manageable. They also take longer to dry, so there's a greater risk of chipping or smudging.

If you're just starting out with at-home polishing, try something airy and light, so that you can get used to the feel and technique of polishing your own nails before moving on to the real tests of skill.

Polishing your toes in challenging colors will help you get used to manipulating these more difficult polishes, so don't hesitate to try them on your toes before switching to using these dramatic colors on your hands.

Under the Stars: hard

whites and clear

White nail polish is usually brought out only to add the tip to a French manicure. But there's so much more you can use it for! An opaque white nail is very chic, with the same versatility as opaque pink except with a little bit more of a twist. And sheer whites can create a beautiful almost nude look that really makes tanned skin pop.

Be wary of using thick, chalky whites—not only do they take forever to dry, but when used as a French tip, they can make your nails and fingers look short and stubby.

Sheer White
It's perfect for an understated French tip, or it can be worn over the entire nail for those allergic to pinks. It's clean and classic, and paints a picture of you as someone who's pulled together, and modern.

Medium White
A good middle tone for an assertive (but not too aggressive and shopping-mall-esque) French manicure, it also works great—edgy and chic—when covering the whole nail. Try it on your toes in the height of summer.

Opaque White
A complete-coverage white, this is the color for those who don't want to give up their bright-white French tips but want to turn classic. It's not translucent, but it keeps the chalkiness at bay and goes on smoothly.

Clearly Perfect
Clear nail polish is the fastest way to highlight beautifully manicured nails. It's always appropriate and lends a very natural, well-groomed air to any set of hands. To me, a woman who chooses clear polish over color always seems confident.

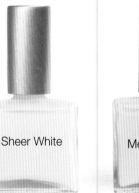

Sheer White

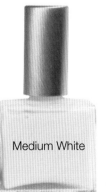

Medium White

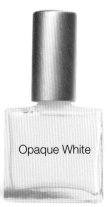

Opaque White

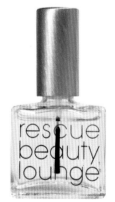

rescue beauty lounge

neutrals

"Neutral" in nail-polish-speak refers to beiges and browns—colors that reflect our natural skin pigmentation. They're low impact, but they can be subtly beautiful, and send a sophisticated, understated vibe. They're a runway staple practically every season.

Sheer Natural

A supersheer true light beige, it's almost a noncolor: no white, no pink. It looks peachy in the bottle, but takes on a beige cast when applied to nails. It's great if you want the sheer, almost-nude look and don't like pinks or whites.

Opaque Natural

The same pigment base as Sheer Natural, this opaque formula is more assertive in its coverage, making it a good choice for feet. It's a classic, sophisticated color— think Catherine Deneuve back in her *Belle de Jour* days.

Opaque Nude

This skin-tone opaque color is used nonstop at all the fashion shows—it's hip, edgy, but still understated. It's like applying foundation to your fingernails, and paints a picture of you as someone who's truly in the know.

Lilac

Lilac? A neutral? You bet it is! Rescue's "Smitten" is the perfect cool neutral, and it's a great way to ease from sheers into colors. It's a subtle spring-fever kind of shade, grown-up yet fun-loving.

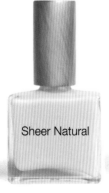
Sheer Natural

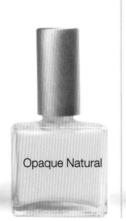
Opaque Natural

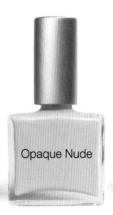
Opaque Nude

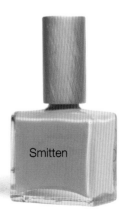
Smitten

pinks

Oh, the pinks—they're the bread and butter of the nail polish industry, and there's also a huge range within the color family. From pale-as-a-whisper sheer to screaming neon, there's a pink for every person, every occasion, and every day!

Clear Pink

A "barely there" color that gives the illusion of a naked, glossy, überhealthy nail plate, this is our most popular color—and the one worn by virtually all the fashion and beauty editors who come into Rescue. You can't go wrong with it: It barely shows chips, it goes with every outfit and every occasion.

Opaque Pink

This is the perfect shade to camouflage discoloration. There's enough opacity to hide any yellow, but it gives the illusion of light, sheer color. It's elegant and versatile enough for a look that exudes powerful femininity. Not too pink . . . not too beige . . . Perfect!

Bubblegum Pink

With it's white base, Rescue's "Lulu" is the classic little girl shade—recast for a sophisticated woman who's a girl at heart. It looks amazing against tanned skin, and the Malibu Barbie brightness will send you right back to a lazy childhood summer vacation.

Pink Shimmer

One of the archaic rules of nail polish that ought to be thrown out the window is that chic women don't wear metallics. Oh, please! A shimmery pink looks amazing on toes, and on fingers it makes you stand out from the crowd of oh-so-predictable pale, glossy pinks.

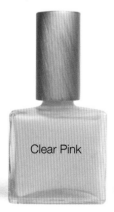

Clear Pink

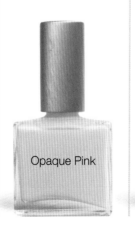

Opaque Pink

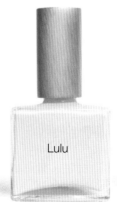

Lulu

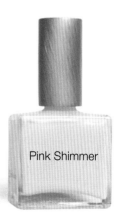

Pink Shimmer

reds

Red is classic. But what's a classic red? If you asked a hundred people, you'd get a hundred different answers. From the socialites of the twenties to the housewives of the fifties to the trendsetters of today, one thing's for sure: Red nails say that you're sexy, powerful, and confident. (Not too long on nail length, please.)

Don't overthink your reds: Does this work well with my skin color? Is it too orange? Too blue? Not blue enough? Try as many reds as you can (including ones you might never think to use) until you find one that works perfectly for you.

Orange-Red

Some might say a color like Rescue's "Chinoise" is too gaudy. And I'll bet those same people say that a Picasso doesn't match their dining room wallpaper. This amazing red is an instant pick-me-up that makes me feel like Diana Vreeland.

Fuchsia Red

A deep pink that reads as red, Rescue's "Cherry Love" is easy to wear. It's a great transitional color—the sultriness of summer fusing with the autumnal warmth of turning leaves.

Classic Red

"Glamourpuss" is a not-too-blue, not-too-orange shade that just oozes old Hollywood glamour. There isn't too much else to say except: Perfect.

Blue-Red

This has a sexiness that will really make your nails shout with its strong statement. When I was wearing our shade around during its testing period, one of my clients cried, "Ji, that red is a killa!" And the name "Killa Red" was born.

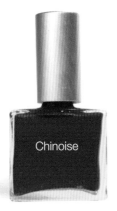
Chinoise

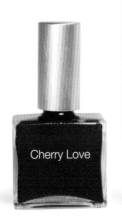
Cherry Love

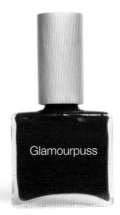
Glamourpuss

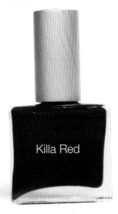
Killa Red

brown reds

The brown-based reds are generally identified as "vampy," which I like to think of as super sexy in an elegant, mysterious, dramatic way. They're a big jump if you're used to wearing only sheer, light colors, but boy oh boy can they ever give you a boost in the sexy-confidence department.

Brown-Burgundy

A perfect mix of rich dark brown and deep burgundy red, Rescue's "Atame" evokes red wine and smooth chocolate. I love this color on the coldest days of winter—it looks great against the pages of the book you're reading while curled up by the fire as a snowstorm rages outside.

Chocolate Brown

I tried for ages to make a perfect deep brown, but it never came out quite right until I added some burgundy to the mix and created "Au Chocolate." The little drop of red keeps the brown tones from becoming too cool. This decadent shade is wildly romantic— urban, sensual, and passionate.

Bordeaux

Inspired by casks of wine and evocative of Paris at the turn of the century, a classic dark red like "Moulin Rouge" is amazingly dark and dangerous. Wear it with confidence . . . and a little bit of caution.

Plum

Our juicy, dark "Drifter" has surprising versatility. It's sexy and edgy for sure, but the purple tone gives it a brightness that makes it everyday-wearable—and it's a great dark color for warmer months. Unique, different— and stunningly beautiful.

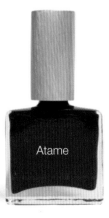
Atame

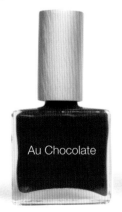
Au Chocolate

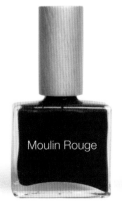
Moulin Rouge

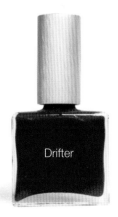
Drifter

cutting-edge colors

These are the ones that make people's eyes pop when they notice your fingers. From dead-body taupey gray to Yves Klein blue to inky black, these colors can be a little intimidating.

But I strongly urge you to take a deep breath and dive in! If after a day of walking around with nails the color of a grassy spring lawn you're still not happy, it's gone with a swipe of a cotton pad. In the meantime, express your-self! You might discover an adventurous side that you never realized existed—live a little!

Grunge
A muddy taupe with lavender undertones and a hint of gray, this might be the last color some people would look at and think "beautiful." But all the trendsetters are knocking down the door for this color, and when it's worn on short nails with a glossy topcoat, it actually winds up looking surprisingly elegant . . . in a hip, edgy way.

Film Noir
The most perfect almost-black aubergine, this deep purple has converted even the

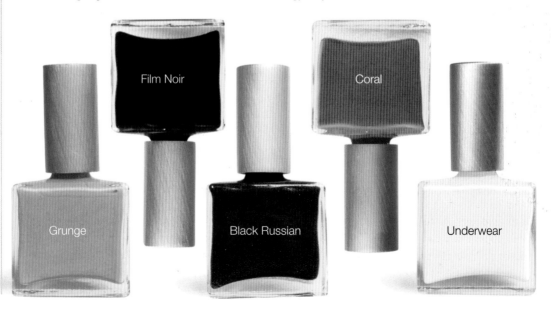

Film Noir

Coral

Grunge

Black Russian

Underwear

shimmer and shine

Most classic colors aren't shiny, but in the past few years, glittery and metallic polishes have been making a much deserved surge to the forefront of chic. From opulent gold to glittering purple to shimmering platinum, the extra punch that a super-shiny polish brings to the table can't be ignored.

Glittery or metallic neutrals are great ways to experiment with polish without moving away from your color comfort zone. Like most out-there shades, though, they work best on short, rounded nails.

While gold, bronze, pink, and red remain the standard-bearers for shimmery

polishes, don't be afraid to branch out in other directions: Rescue's "Leila," a metallic lilac, and "Pippa," a rich gold-pink, are unexpected hues that take your fingertips to a whole new level.

Due to the presence of a shiny mineral called mica in their pigment, metallic polish jobs last a lot longer than nonmetallics. The mica clings for dear life to your nail plate, and can be incredibly difficult to take off. So if you're wearing a metallic, take care to apply your base coat properly so that when it's time to take the color off, it comes off!

most aesthetically conservative to the dark side! Wear it on short nails—if your tips are like talons, it'll look cartoonish. But on short nails it makes you look artsy, sexy, and confident.

Black Russian
A true black with ruby-red microglitter, this polish reads as black, red, purple, or glittery, depending on the light. It's one of the rare dark shades that actually has depth, so it's a surprisingly easy color to wear . . . and people know it! This color barely stays in stock—every time a new shipment comes in it flies off the shelves.

Coral
That's right, your grandma's favorite shade is a cutting-edge color, not because there's anything so unexpected about the shade itself, but because it's gone so far into the realm of granny that it seems as if its reputation might never recover. Not so! A true coral doesn't say old lady, it says Palm Springs, St-Tropez, Rio—teeny bikinis and deep tans. Stay away from shades that are more salmon than pink, and wear this rich, luscious, ripe color with confidence.

Underwear
This "neon" white grew out of a fashion-week need for layered color. Top this überbright, überwhite shade with any sheer color and prepare to be amazed by the backlighting effect. Or wear it alone for something that blazes mod from miles away—as chic as black, but even more unexpected and contemporary.

caring for your polish

Whether it's a neon pink from the 99-cent bin, or you dropped a day's pay on the latest of-the-moment designer enamel, your polish deserves to be treated right. With the proper care and storage, you can help lengthen its life and maintain its quality. No one wants to reach for her favorite go-to shade, minutes before needing to be out the door, only to find that it's a gloopy, separated mess!

The standard shelf life for a bottle of nail polish is two years, but with the right attention to detail you can help it last even longer. Here are some guidelines for keeping your lacquers luscious!

With Each Use

Each time you use your polish, take a few seconds to prep it for next time. Before replacing the brush-cap after use, clean the lip of the bottle with a paper towel dipped in

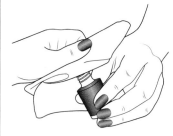

nail polish remover. (Don't use cotton balls—they'll just make the bottle all fuzzy!) This not only makes it easier for you to open the bottle the next time you want to use

this color, it also makes an airtight seal that prolongs the life of your polish.

Storing Between Uses

Nail polish is a complicated chemical concoction that's developed and tested to be used—and stored—within certain ranges of temperature. If there's one thing I've learned through the process of developing my own polish line, it's not to mess with those parameters! Nail polish should be stored at room temperature, avoiding extremes of hot or cold. I'm not sure who it was who started the rumor that storing nail polish in the refrigerator

is a good idea, but it's not: It's a huge mistake. The enamel might appear smoother at first application, but as the polish warms to your body temperature the ingredients in the polish will begin to change, and there will be bubbling and stringing—not the most glamorous look for your manicure.

While bottles of polish can look glamorous clustered on a countertop or on a tray on top of a vanity, watch out for the sun: Some colors are susceptible to fading, so it can't hurt to keep your collection of colors in a drawer, an opaque pouch, or a chic box.

in the buff: naked nails

A natural buff—polish-free nails that are shined to a high-gloss finish—is the most basic, classic look for absolutely everyone. It works on both fingers and toes, and takes the buffing that you do in the basic At-Home Manicure (page 39) and At-Home Pedicure (page 57) to a whole new level. It works on everyone: whatever your nail shape, your nail length, your personal style—even your gender! And if you're a polisher, buffing your nails is like priming a canvas: Especially if you have deep ridges, it creates the perfect even surface on which to create your masterpiece.

For the average person, once a month is the ideal frequency for buffing to create and maintain a healthy look. (If you have weak or brittle nails, downscale that to once every four to six months. And don't forget to take vitamins to build up your nail strength!)

It couldn't be easier to acquire the tools for getting a set of perfectly buffed nails. You absolutely need to get a three-sided file, which is readily available at any drugstore or beauty-supply store. This type of file allows you a tremendous degree of control over the amount of pressure you're placing on the nail.

A three-sided file has—surprise, surprise—three different grades of file along its sides. The toughest is used to sand down the top layer of the nails, the medium grade evens out the first layer, and then the smooth side seals the nail plate with a high-gloss finish. As with all nonmetal tools, it's good for one use only.

mise en place

Tools

☐ Three-sided buffing file

Supplies

☐ Cotton pads or cotton swabs

Products

☐ Nail polish remover

☐ Hand cream or cuticle oil

1 If you're wearing nail polish, soak a cotton pad in remover and take off all the polish, using firm, even strokes. Use a cotton swab to get into the corners and along the cuticle of your nails. Whether or not you were wearing nail polish, dip a cotton swab or soak a cotton pad in polish remover and swipe across the surface of your bare nail to remove any oil residue. The entire nail should look dull and matte once it's fully cleaned.

2 Using the roughest side of the three-sided file, gently file the entire top surface of your nail. It will look rough and white—don't worry! Don't overlook the corners and edge.

3 Repeat the process using the medium side of the file: Gently move the file over the entire surface of the nail, lightly brushing off any accumulating debris.

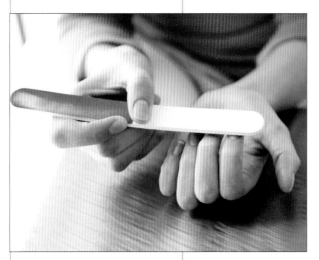

4 Using long, smooth, quick strokes, file down the surface of the nail using the smoothest side of the file. This should remove any

The three-sided file is the only tool you need.

remaining roughness or imperfection. If you're planning to apply polish, now is when you should start the application process (see page 77).

5 If you're not planning to follow your buff with an application of nail polish, rub oil or cuticle cream onto your cuticles, massage hand cream onto the rest of your hand, and admire your naked—and beautiful—nails!

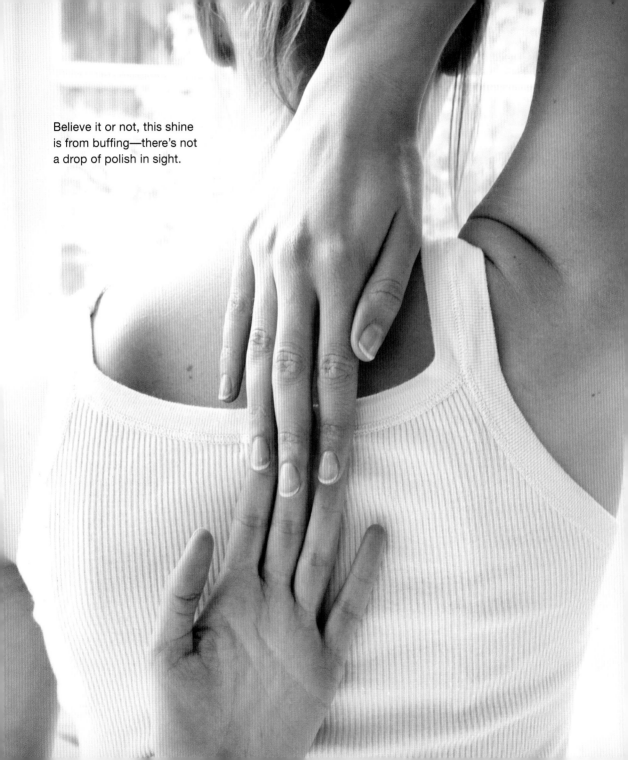

Believe it or not, this shine
is from buffing—there's not
a drop of polish in sight.

My mantra: Treat your hands the way you treat your face—with lots of attention and the utmost care.

the skin you're in

It should be clear by now that there's more to a manicure than shaping and polishing your nails—it's just as much about your hands. There's a reason that hand models are among the highest paid in the business. A perfect set of hands is a rare thing to come by, and is even harder to maintain. As with all models, though, hand models don't come by their perfection without effort. They have to work to make sure that their hands are in perfect, photographable condition at all times.

I've met my share of hand models throughout my career, and they are known for being obsessive about ensuring that their hands are absolutely perfect. The rumors are true: They *do* wear gloves and long sleeves all the time—while eating dinner, while sleeping, while at the beach—to protect their skin. And they're flat-out religious about moisturization and protection.

We don't have to go to the extremes that hand models do (and we can be grateful that we don't have to keep our hands in gloves 24/7!), but there's a lesson to be learned from their obsessive maintenance. Our hands tell the story of a life's worth of wear and tear, but with only a little effort we can prevent and even reverse damage done by age, sun, environment, and neglect. Dry cuticles, age spots, rough skin—there are dozens of ways your hands can be less than perfect. Fortunately, for every problem, there's an effective and oftentimes easy solution.

aging hands

be prepared

One of the chicest women I've ever met owned dozens and dozens of handbags, and in every one she kept a quarter, a twenty-dollar bill, and a Chanel lipstick in her favorite shade. I just wish she'd added hand cream! I keep a travel-size bottle of hand cream in every bag I own, so I don't have to worry about whether I've remembered to transfer it along with my wallet, cell phone, and everything else.

Age spots and crepelike skin are the hallmarks of aging hands, and they seem to show up practically overnight. In fact, the most common complaint I hear from my clients is that they wish their hands didn't show age so suddenly. But the truth is that hands age as gradually and steadily as the rest of your body—much like your face, your hands are a prime place for the passage of time to reveal itself. Unfortunately, most people don't start treating the signs of aging until they've already presented themselves. You can help slow the process—or reverse some damage that's already been done—by paying particular attention to the products you use to maintain your hands.

Most women know the antiaging drill when it comes to their faces: Moisturize obsessively. Start using antiwrinkle cream when you're in your twenties. Drink plenty of water. Get plenty of sleep. Alpha peels, beta peels, microdermabrasion, creams and makeups infused with the highest SPF money can buy . . . we pull all the stops when it comes to keeping our faces looking young (and it works!). But what's the point of having a luminous, youthful face if our hands give it all away?

Here's the answer: Treat your hands the way you treat your face. I often get looked at as if I have an alien head when I insist that our clients use the same products for their hands that they use for the delicate skin on their cheeks and forehead. But heavy-duty moisturizers, spot-fading peels and toners, and gentle cleansers will help smooth and plump your skin, while moisturizer with a high SPF will help slow further damage. Maintaining a routine is key: Just as you religiously apply your antiwrinkle

the many uses of moisturizer

Hand cream, face cream, body cream. Whatever the label calls it, this emollient is a magical multi-purpose tool. Not only will it rehydrate parched skin, but a little dab of moisturizer can serve as:

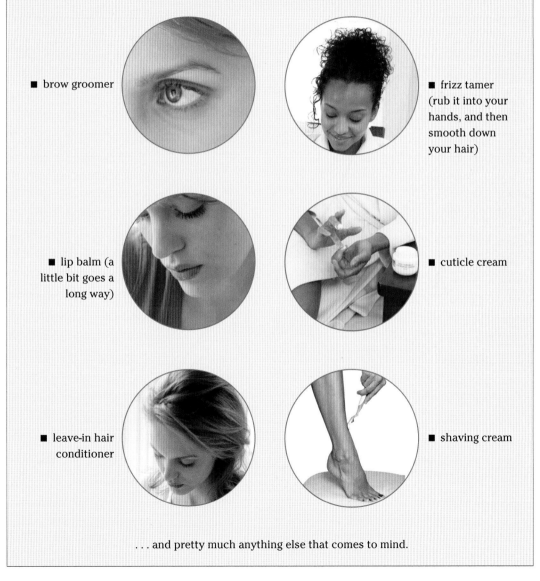

- brow groomer

- frizz tamer (rub it into your hands, and then smooth down your hair)

- lip balm (a little bit goes a long way)

- cuticle cream

- leave-in hair conditioner

- shaving cream

. . . and pretty much anything else that comes to mind.

where to keep moisturizer

At work: *right next to your phone,* so that every time you take or make a call, you're reminded to moisturize.

At home: *next to the bed, so it's the first* thing you see when you wake up in the morning and the last thing you see when you go to sleep at night.

Next to every sink in your house: *kitchen,* bathrooms, workroom, laundry room, garage. Anywhere your hands can get wet, you can lose moisture. Be on your guard!

Anywhere else you can think of: Buy little bottles of hand cream

(or dispense your favorite moisturizer into travel-size containers) and stash them everywhere: your pocketbook, your computer bag, your gym bag, the glove compartment in your car, the gardening shed, the pocket in your baby's stroller, your schoolbag, your makeup bag . . . you get the idea!

face cream each night before bed, you should religiously apply antiwrinkle cream to the backs of your hands and fingers.

Preventing or slowing the signs of age on your hands is simply a matter of extending your face-care regimen to your digits. Take a little extra of your glycolic acid peel or AHA lotion, and rub it into the backs of your hands. Use the same SPF moisturizer you'd use on your face (most facial moisturizing formulas are gentler than general body moisturizers), and be as wary of keeping the sun off your hands, via gloves or longer sleeves, as you are about keeping the sun off your face.

Once the spots and wrinkles have started appearing, it's tough to turn back the clock and make them disappear entirely (at least not without resorting to expensive cosmetic treatments). You can wish as hard as you like, but the signs of aging will always get worse—not better—unless you take steps to alleviate them.

If you're using a particularly dense facial moisturizer or cream, you might want to apply it to your hands only at night. During the day, you use your hands more than you use your face (not too many women I know use their noses and cheeks to type on their BlackBerries!), so sleep time is the perfect chance for your resting hands to absorb some much needed nutrients.

working hands

Your hands tell a story: your family history (I have my grandfather's hands, wrinkly and red) and your life history (every cut, scar, burn, or scrape). We use our hands all day, every day. Whether it's shuffling papers or cutting wood, our hands are the tools we use to interact with the world. In my long history with other people's hands, I've learned how to tell what they do with their lives by the story their hands tell me: chefs, gardeners, ladies of leisure whose biggest decision is where to have lunch. It's all revealed in your hands, and you should be proud of what the wear and tear on your hands reveals about who you are. But odds are good that you don't need to show as much of it as you do. The tips on the following pages can help you adapt your job or hobby to preserve your hands' health and youthfulness, without giving anything up.

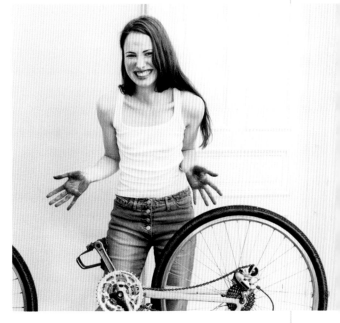

Getting your hands dirty doesn't mean treating them badly!

Kitchen Hands

A serious dedication to cooking produces beautiful meals, but it leaves your hands anything *but* beautiful. At every turn, there's another threat to the well-being of your hands and nails—from wet sinks to blisteringly hot stoves to sharp knives to abrasive ingredients. The kitchen is a minefield! But with a little attention to detail, it's possible to keep your hands as smooth as your famous hollandaise. As it is to other problem environments, moisturization is a key element to preserving your hands. If you're worried about mixing a chemical-based moisturizer with something you'll end up eating, moisturize with a little bit of olive oil or butter. They're just as good as hand cream!

Cutting and Chopping

Here, a good offense is the best defense: Work on your knife skills! Whether you practice on your own or take a class, becoming comfortable with your tools will help minimize slips and cuts. Nothing mars a beautiful finger like a long, unsightly gash.

And it's not just knives that have dangerous edges: vegetable peelers, mandolins, cheese graters, scissors, zesters, blenders, food processors . . . sometimes it can seem like there's something sharp everywhere you turn. The best way to avoid hurting yourself is to be conscientious and cautious with all kitchen operations: Use finger guards with any machines or tools that call for them, never reach into a machine while it's still running, and store your knives, peelers, and graters in places where you won't accidentally brush against them when reaching into a drawer or onto a shelf.

If, despite your perfect knife skills, you do happen to cut yourself, be responsible: Stop what you're doing and wash the cut immediately, and apply antibiotic ointment *whether or not the cut looks like it needs it.* Besides being effective antiseptics, these ointments (Neosporin in particular) also contain powerful moisturizers that

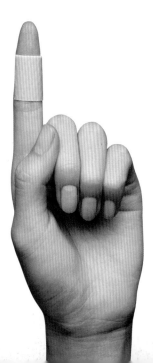

Be sure to bandage any cuts—no matter how small.

The kitchen can be
a dangerous place
for your hands.

The fix?

You guessed it: Moisturize!

help your skin heal more quickly and with less of a chance of scarring. Bandage your cut and keep it dry with a latex glove or a finger guard (a finger-only latex sleeve, available at most drugstores).

Steam and Water

Whatever good steam does for your face by opening and flushing out your pores, it *doesn't* do it for your hands. Steam is drying: As your hands dry after they've been immersed in steam, they give off more moisture than you want them to. This can be counteracted by wearing rubber or silicone gloves while dealing with steam and hot liquids, or by remembering to moisturize soon after contact.

It's not only the hot stuff that has a drying effect, though: Water at any temperature leeches moisture as it evaporates from your skin, so even rinsing vegetables or kneading a moist dough can dry you out. The fix? You guessed it: Moisturize!

Burns

A real occupational hazard for the serious chef, burns sear your skin, leaving it red and shiny. There's a lot you can do to prevent burns in the first place: Wear oven mitts, invest in heatproof silicone pot-handle covers, and be careful when working around open flames or hot metal, water, or oil. Always pay attention!

If you do wind up with a burn—and it happens to all of us!—it helps to be prepared ahead of time: Have burn cream, bandages, and a clean towel in an easily accessible place in the kitchen for making a cold compress. Keep an aloe vera plant in the kitchen (you can find one at most any garden-supply store, and at many grocery stores, as well). The plants have thick leaves that ooze a nutrient-rich liquid that is a phenomenal all-purpose burn salve, moisturizer, facial mask, and skin protector.

If you do slip up and hurt yourself, first assess the degree of your burn. If there is immediate blistering, or the skin looks raw, immediately get medical attention. For mild burns that don't require medical attention, run icy cold water over your hand, gently pat it dry, and then *immediately* apply burn cream or aloe. Cover the burn securely with a loosely applied clean bandage.

If you get a quick searing burn—you accidentally touch a hot stove or get a little boiling water on your finger—you'll want to attend to it right away: Apply burn cream or aloe. The moisture and nutrients help protect your hurt skin against abrasion. Follow with ice or a cold compress.

Unwanted Odors

Mincing garlic, filleting a fish, emulsifying a vinaigrette . . . the kitchen is full of delicious ingredients whose less-than-delicious scents linger on your fingers long after the prep work is done. Get rid of unwanted odors by washing your hands thoroughly with warm water and a gentle cleanser to get rid of any surface oils. Dry your hands completely and then wash them again. If the odor persists, rub some salt and lemon juice into your hands and then rinse it off.

Protection While Cooking

Even if disaster doesn't strike, there are little ways to protect your hands while you're cooking. Olive oil, butter, or any other fat makes a wonderful moisturizer. When you're rubbing butter over a chicken or oiling a baking pan, take a second to rub some of the lipid into your hands (though be wary of getting your palms and fingers too slippery to grip your equipment). When you're slicing lemons or using lemon juice, rub it into your fingernails—the citric acid helps make your nails whiter. And be careful not to move your hands too quickly from the deep cold of the freezer to the serious heat over the stovetop: The rapid change in temperature can cause your hands to dry out very quickly.

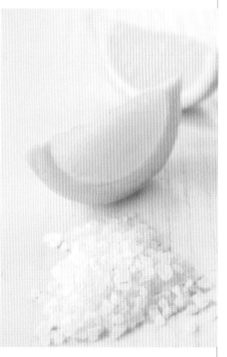

Lemon and salt:
Nature's deodorizers.

Gardening gloves are the chicest accessory to protect your most valuable tools.

Gardening Hands

It's wonderful to garden, isn't it? Becoming one with the earth, bringing forth flowers and vegetables to enjoy and share with friends is a satisfying, soothing delight. Whether you're a lifelong gardening devotee or a one-day-a-year wonder, it can run a number on your hands if you're not careful.

There are two rules when it comes to your hands and gardening: First, always wear gloves. Not only do they protect your hands from scrapes, cuts, and stains, they're also the absolute best protection against the sun. Most people are tremendously conscientious when it comes to protecting their faces, necks, and shoulders against the harmful UV rays that are always present (even on overcast days!): They wear hats and long sleeves, and lavish their exposed skin with sunblock. But many gardeners forget that the skin on their hands is as sensitive to the sun as their faces are—if not more so—and deserves at least as much protection. When my clients ask me if they should be wearing a high SPF hand cream when working in the garden, I tell them not to worry about it—because they should be wearing gloves instead!

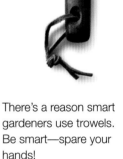

There's a reason smart gardeners use trowels. Be smart—spare your hands!

The second rule when it comes to gardening is this: Your hands are NOT tools. It's tempting to dig with your fingers, but don't! Don't dig, don't rake, don't pinch off buds or twist off leaves. There are wonderful tools that have been designed for just these purposes, and incorporating them into your gardening routine can help save your hands, so that once you go inside and wash off the dirt, your skin and nails are lovely enough to take you out to a black-tie gala.

Glove-free Gardening

For all that I insist on using gardening gloves all the time, I know that there are times when it's easier to have your hands and fingers free. If you're doing delicate work for which gloves get in the way, there are ways to take preventative steps that, while not quite as effective as full-on gloves, are a good way to be conscious of protecting your hands and nails. First and foremost, make sure to apply sunblock with a high SPF to your forearms and hands—all over! Reapply it every 20 or so minutes, and try if at all possible to limit the amount of glove-free gardening that you do during the time of strongest sunlight, which is between 10 A.M. and 3 P.M.

Office Hands

I know what you're thinking: Working in an office is the *best* thing I can do for my hands! I'm not outside under the sun, I'm not near hot stoves or heavy equipment or toxic chemicals. Why do office hands need special care? The truth is that the wear on your hands that happens with a desk job is real, and it's insidious—it happens gradually, until one day you look down at your chapped, dull hands and barely recognize them.

Paper is, bar none, **the worst enemy** of moisturized skin.

What's the culprit? One word: paper. Paper is, bar none, the worst enemy of moisturized skin: It sucks up every drop from already parched cuticles and fingertips. Add to that the stresses of typing, gripping pens and pencils, and drying, climate-controlled air and your cuticles are probably so dry you could practically crack them off with your newly brittle fingernails. (Don't!)

Maintaining your hands at the office is a simple matter of keeping moisturizer at your desk and using it. *Often.*

To help preserve strength and beauty in your fingernails, don't use them as tools. Don't use the tips to dig out staples, to dial the phone, or to type on a calculator or computer. Don't lick your fingertips when you turn over a piece of paper. All of these lead to weakening and dryness.

Those piles of paper leach
moisture right out of your skin.

hands in extreme conditions

If you come into frequent contact with harsh chemicals (the kind found in industrial-strength cleaning agents, for instance, or in some beauty products such as hair dye), if your hands are wet for long periods of the day, or if they are frequently exposed to strong heat or serious cold, you'll need to take particular care to help keep your skin looking supple and smooth.

This deep conditioner for your hands should leave them feeling packed with moisture, and will help soften the dry, hardened skin that can come from prolonged exposure to extreme conditions. As often as you can—daily, if possible—give your hands this intensive "masque" treatment.

You'll need:
- heavy moisturizing cream
- plastic wrap

Slather your hands and forearms with the moisturizing cream, and snugly (but not too snugly) wrap them in plastic wrap. Keep wrapping up your forearm, pressing the plastic to seal it down. Pretend this is a spa body wrap for just your hand. Leave the wrapping on for at least 10 minutes—watch TV, listen to music, or just daydream—and then remove the plastic and discard it.

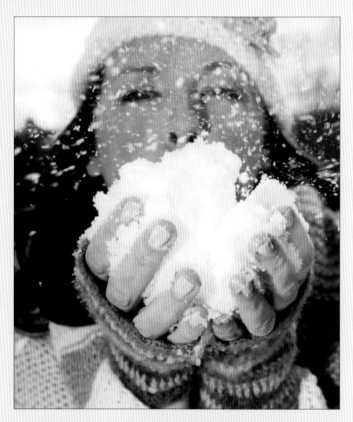

If you can't be without the use of your hands for 10 minutes, put on a thick layer of moisturizer under a pair of plastic gloves (latex works well, though of course don't use them if you have a latex allergy). Leave the gloves on for 10 minutes or more, and then remove and discard them.

Moisturize, Moisturize, Moisturize!

It's probably clear to you by now that almost every problem can be solved with a generous application of lipids. It's the one-word answer that I give to every single person who comes into Rescue and complains about the skin on her hands. No matter how awful, how coarse, how flaky, the answer is: MOISTURIZE. A couple of pumps of hand cream will snap even the worst skin right back into short-term fighting shape, and a dedicated daily moisturizing regimen can pretty much work miracles.

To boost your hand care regimen—whether you do manual labor, are trying to stave off the signs of age, or are simply interested in maintaining your hands' beauty—start keeping a bottle of moisturizer or hand cream with a pump top next to each sink in your home. Hydrate after every washing, as well as whenever your hands start to feel dry or tight. I've tried this out on my friends, on my clients, and on myself, and the evidence is overwhelming: Hands that are kept hydrated all day long look youthful, smoother, and more supple. Which is the goal, after all.

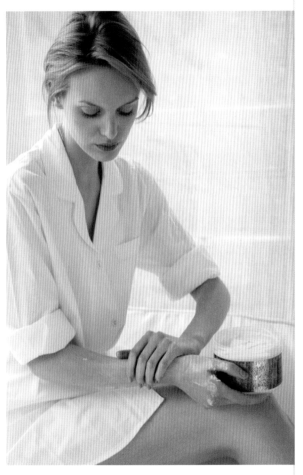

Lotion, body butter, emollient . . . whatever you call it, use it!

Some people complain that their moisturizer is too greasy to use as frequently as I've prescribed, and that they can't type on the computer or shuffle paperwork with greasy hands. Come on—this is a silly excuse! Either blot off the greasy residue with a tissue (just like lipstick, lotion can be blotted), or switch to a less greasy formula. There's no excuse for not sticking to your routine!

Don't you wish all
your problems were
this easy to fix?

the imperfect nail: troubleshooting

For all the time and energy we invest in making our nails, hands, and feet beautiful, some things are just beyond our control . . . or are they? For virtually every problem, pain, or imperfection, there's a way to alleviate it and help keep it from recurring. It's just a matter of knowing what's normal and what's not—and what to do about it.

With all the use we get out of our hands, it's amazing that they're not *more* flawed. But we've still got plenty to work with. Whether it's weakness, splitting, ridges, spots, discoloration, or simple dissatisfaction with their shape, it seems like everyone has found a flaw or two in her fingernails. Too often I've met people who are willing to live with those flaws. But it's a simple matter to make some small changes that will have big effects! Beyond basic filing and moisturizing, sometimes we need a little extra TLC.

And then there are the girls downstairs. To many of us, our feet are a complete mystery—maybe because they're way down on the floor. But from jagged toenails to rough calluses, our heels, soles, and toes are worthy of just as much attention as our hands. After all, we're not walking around on our hands all day in four-inch heels or hard, tight gloves. Our poor feet deserve a break, too!

types of problems

the gelatin effect

Here's an enduring nail care myth: The best way to strengthen your nails is to eat gelatin—a gelling agent used in cooking, and the primary ingredient in that jiggly, wiggly dessert we all grew up with. Does it work? Yes and no.

Consuming enough protein is essential when it comes to strengthening your nails, and gelatin is a pure protein derived from animal collagen. However, it hasn't been proven to be particularly more effective than any other type of protein—consuming meat, vegetable, or soy protein will strengthen your nails just as effectively.

Feed Your Weak Nails

"Why do I have such weak nails?" wail so many of my clients. You might as well ask why you have brown hair or why you've got a dusting of freckles on your arms. The strength of your nails is by and large a product of good old DNA. Look at your siblings, parents, cousins, children: Do they have weak nails, too? If so, close the book. We've solved the mystery of your weak nails, and the only solution is to keep them strong by adding a layer of strengthening base coat and polish.

If your family's nails aren't weak, or if you're convinced there's got to be more to it, take a look at what you're feeding your nails. And by "feeding" I don't mean the lotions and oils you're rubbing on, I mean actual food. Like your hair, your nails are made primarily of keratin, which is a fibrous protein. And just as your diet can affect the lustrousness of your hair or the clarity of your skin, a balanced intake of vitamins, proteins, and calcium will help strengthen your fingernails. Many of my clients are very disciplined about maintaining a certain weight, and I can always tell the ones who take it too far—whose regimented diets are veering dangerously toward unhealthy eating disorders—by their nails: brittle, thin, and weak.

I'm sure that no matter how young you are, whenever you go to the doctor, you're reminded to up your calcium intake to fend off osteoporosis. And I'm sure that, just like me, you put it out of your head as soon as you leave the office. Osteoporosis? It's so far in the future, who wants to drink an extra glass of milk now? Well,

You are what you eat:
Healthy, beautiful foods lead
to healthy, beautiful nails.
And don't forget to take your
vitamins!

If you can't stand the notion of waiting for discolored nails to clear up on their own, there are a few at-home remedies that can affect the color right away.

■ Dip the bristles of a nail brush or old toothbrush into hydrogen peroxide, and gently scrub your nails.

■ Squeeze the juice from a quarter of a lemon onto each hand's nails, and scrub well with a nail brush or old toothbrush.

■ Apply dabs of oxygen cream (available at beauty supply stores; if you can't find it, you can use any brightening or whitening facial cream) to each fingernail like a mask. Leave it on for five minutes, and then gently buff off with a buffing block or disk, using an X motion (see page 47).

listen up: If spending your future hunched over isn't enough to motivate you, know that a high-calcium diet can have an almost immediate effect on the health of your nails. If you don't do it for your bones, do it for your fingernails. Consider the added bone density a nice little bonus! Along with a diet rich in calcium, make sure that you're getting a balance of other vitamins, especially vitamin E.

Last, if you have weak nails: Don't fight nature. The best way to keep your nails healthy and attractive is to keep them short and well groomed, with rounded corners that are supported by your nail bed—no overhang!

Not-So-Mellow Yellow: What Happened to My Nail Color?

Nail polish can do more than just strengthen your nails—it can also mask discoloration, which is one of the ways your nails give a cry for help. If you're the sort of person who wears nail polish all the time, think about it. When do you give your nails a chance to breathe? For most of us, it's just between taking one color off and putting the next one on: twenty minutes, tops. And heavily pigmented colors—applied improperly, without a base coat—can seep into the nail itself, discoloring the keratin.

It's not hard to prevent discoloration:

■ Always—and I mean *always*—use base coat on a well-prepped nail. It's tempting to skip this step at home, since you can't see the base coat once the manicure is done, but it's critical. It helps prevent chipping by bonding the polish to the nail. Equally important, it provides a protective layer between the pigment in the polish and your nail.

■ Rotate your colors. If you favor dark colors with heavy pigmentation, switch it up and wear a light color for one week each month.

■ If your discoloration is severe, trim your nails short to promote new growth, and go cold turkey from nail polish for one week. Try a buffed nail (see page 99), if your nails are strong enough. It's a great cleanup.

If it's your polish—not your nails—that appears yellow, don't worry. All it means is that your topcoat, which protects the polish, has worn off, and the pigment has oxidized. This is most common on a sunny day at the beach or in the park. Not only does the sunlight itself promote oxidation, but many products—including hair chemicals, face products containing alpha hydroxy or glycolic acids, detergents, and sunblock and other products with SPF—can lead to a quicker breakdown of the topcoat. Feel free to reapply.

Ridges

One of the most common complaints among my clients is ridged nails, which can be caused by any number of factors: hormones, genes, or some sort of behavior that affects the surface of the nail. There are as many types of ridges as there are colors of nail polish, but they fall into a few broad categories.

If your nails are ridged but are otherwise strong, the ridges most likely take the form of a ripply irregularity in the surface of the nail. These ridges are a piece of cake to take care of: Simply smooth the surface of the nail with a buffing block or disk, using an *X*-shaped motion like the one described on (page 47). The ridges will come back as the nails grow out, but you can always buff them away again.

In weak nails, ridges are "furrows," ridges from root to tip that split and break once they grow past the end of the nail bed. In this case, there isn't much choice beyond wearing your nails short enough to keep the tips from splitting. A binding agent—

ridge fillers

Ridge fillers are basically a dense version of base coat, which settle into the ridges and create the appearance of a more uniform nail surface. They're helpful for shallow ridges, as are any base coats or polishes, but won't cure anything. It's a tool, not a solution.

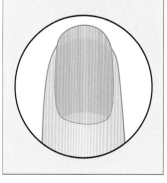

ridges and polish

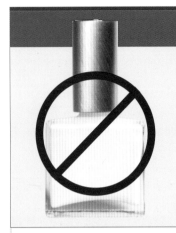

If your ridges are severe, avoid nail polishes with a white base: opaque whites, pinks, and pastels. These colors accentuate ridges, and applying enough polish to hide them will create a thick, gloppy coat of polish that won't look anything close to attractive and will take hours to dry. While reds or dark colors work just fine, my favorite choice for visually smoothing the nail is something light, sheer, and classic.

even a simple coat of clear nail polish—is a perfect coat of armor: It will help reinforce the nail and offset its propensity for splitting. Avoid buffing the top of your nails, since weak nails need all the structure they can get.

A habit of rubbing your fingertips across the top of your nail plate, from stress or boredom, can cause ridges, too. It's not as bad a habit as biting your nails, and (curiously) men tend to do it more than women do. Instead of the usual cure for a woman—wearing a coat of nail polish to protect the surface of the nail—men can do a full buff, smoothing out the ridges and moisturizing the nails to help break the habit.

If your nails have been healthy and beautiful all your life and then ridges suddenly appear, check with your physician. It can be caused by a nutritional imbalance or a hormonal fluctuation, or it can be a side effect of certain medications.

Splitsville?

There is nothing more annoying than a split or broken nail—and often there's nothing more painful, either. It happens to the best of us: an errant table corner, a too-hard tap on a cell phone keypad, a fast rip of tape off a box, or even (tsk-tsk!) an aggressive nail-biting spree. Whether your nails are weak and prone to splitting or you have perfectly healthy nails that you just so happen to occasionally use as power tools, you'll need to learn how to take care of a split.

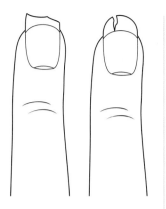

If one of your nails breaks (left) or splits (right)—it's time to start fresh with all of them.

■ If the split is just on the tip (it doesn't reach the nail bed), use your clippers to trim off both sides of the broken nail, and then file the tip down evenly. If there's a disparity between the length of your newly filed nail and the others, take a deep breath and trim those, too. Nails always look more elegant when they're even, rather than at irregular lengths.

■ If the split goes all the way to your nail bed, trim the tip to the edge of your finger and then wash your hands with antibacterial soap. Once your hands are fully dry, go to your first aid kit and apply Neosporin to the damaged nail, followed by an adhesive bandage to protect from further damage. Wear bandages for several days, changing them whenever they get loose, wet, or dirty, and always reapply Neosporin when changing the bandage.

White Spots!

Everyone gets them. Everyone freaks out about them. And the reasons we're given for them are seemingly infinite. It's a calcium deficiency? It's a zinc deficiency? It's a sign that you're unhealthy or not exercising or getting old? Nope, sorry, none of the above. Here's the truth. It is, basically, a bruise: a mark that appears when you bang your nails slightly, often without even knowing it, and disrupt the new nail tissue that's forming in the matrix. Let it grow out, and treat it like it's just a normal part of your nail.

Of course, if your white spot is very large, is raised up or indented, or in any other way seems abnormal—have a doctor check it out. Better safe than sorry!

homemade wraps

If your nails are long, your split doesn't extend past the nail bed, and you simply must *save it,
do an at-home wrap—basically a cast for your broken nail. How? This just might be the best-kept
secret of the nail industry: facial tissue plus nail glue, a specially formulated glue sold at most
drugstores and beauty supply stores.*

1. *Cut a square of one-ply facial tissue about the size of
your nail. Use the nonmoisturized kind, and separate out a
layer if all you have are multi-ply.* **2.** *Place the tissue over the
split.* **3.** *Drip the nail glue onto it one drop at a time, letting it
soak into the fiber of the tissue and adhere it to your nail. Do it
slowly—it should look like the tissue is melting into your nail—
and don't use too much glue.* **4.** *Let it dry, and buff it smooth
with a block or disk. Voila!*

BOTTOMS UP:

foot therapy

Does the Shape of My Toenails Matter?

Absolutely! Having toenails that are irregularly shaped, too long, or too short can lead to pinching or rubbing when you wear shoes.

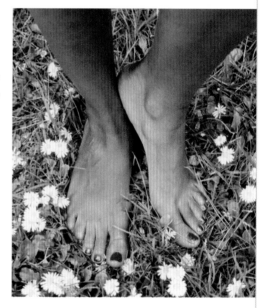

And when your foot hurts, everything hurts. Just remember what it's like to have a fresh blister or to hobble around with a newly stubbed toe. With careful attention to the grooming of your toenails, you can avoid the pitfalls that lead to discomfort—particularly ingrown toenails.

I used to suffer horribly from ingrown toenails, especially on my big toes, and I know the whole routine. I'd grab nippers and cut out the corners of the nail that was digging into my poor skin, and then dig around and get out as much of the dead skin in that corner as I could. I was addicted to this vicious cycle. I dug, I bled, over and over . . . It wasn't until my podiatrist yelled at me to STOP! that I realized I was doing more harm than good.

So, learn from one former sufferer's personal experience. Here's how to break the cycle of picking and clipping:

■ Never ever cut the corners of your toenail. It just leaves room for the skin in the corners of your nail bed to grow in, which makes growing out your nails even more painful—they have to push through the skin to break free of the nail bed. Let your nails grow out. This might take a few weeks, and the first three or four days might be torturously painful. If you get through it once, though, you won't ever have to go through it again (at least, as long as you're diligent about the rest of these steps!).

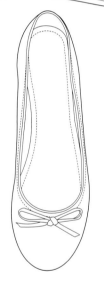

■ Wear shoes with a lower heel and a toe box that doesn't pinch your toes together. If you do have to give in to fashion and break out the four-inch stilettos, select rounded toes, and keep your time standing— and especially walking—to a minimum.

■ When you're wearing closed-toed shoes, keep your toenails trimmed. Long toenails in an enclosed space means you're inviting trouble.

■ Trim your toenails straight across. No rounded corners, no fancy shapes.

■ Stop cutting the corner of your nails, stop digging out dead skin. Let your nails grow on their own.

If you find that your ingrown toenails are inordinately painful, or the skin around your toenail looks red and raised, don't try to fix it yourself. Do the smart thing and get it checked out by a doctor.

Callus Malice

Poor calluses get such a bad rap. A callus is an extra layer of thick skin that develops wherever there's a point of serious pressure, and it forms for one reason only: to protect you. Haven't you noticed that they show up on the spots on your feet that experience the most stress? The outside of your heels, the center of the ball of your foot, and the outside of your big toe: three weight-bearing areas that also tend to rub against the insides of your shoes with every step.

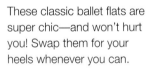

These classic ballet flats are super chic—and won't hurt you! Swap them for your heels whenever you can.

Under no circumstances should you use a callus shaver (also called a credo knife), which in most states is actually illegal. This little tool looks like a miniature cheese shaver, and it's for slicing off your skin. If the thought of basically taking a knife to yourself isn't enough to put you off, consider this: After you slice off your calluses, your skin simply reforms them. And when they come back, they tend to be thicker and more uneven than before, which leads to cracking.

Calluses themselves aren't bad, but accepting that you've got them doesn't give you an excuse to let them go ungroomed. There should be no reason yours are so dry that they crack. Moisturize your calluses as much as, if not more than, you do the rest of your foot, and run a foot file over them every time you're in the shower. Let them protect you—it's their job!

That's So Corny

After a couple of years of battling your size 8 feet into those darling sample-sale Louboutins (they're a 6½—that's practically the same thing!), you've probably noticed little hard lumps of skin developing on the tops of your toes. These are corns, and they're nothing to worry about.

Like a callus, a corn is simply a layer of thick skin that forms in response to pressure or friction in concentrated areas. In fact, calluses and corns are medically identical, but while calluses generally refer to thickened skin on the sides and bottom of the foot (or anywhere else on the body), a corn is specifically a callus that forms on the tops or sides of the toes.

You can prevent corns from forming by wearing well-fitting shoes and avoiding tight toe boxes (and sample sales!). But if the damage is already done (and believe me, I can relate to giving in to the siren call of a dreamy pair of perfect pumps), you can soften and smooth corns by keeping them exfoliated and well moisturized.

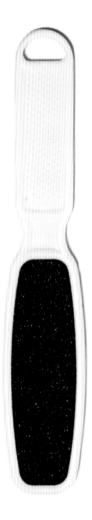

A foot file is the superstar of exfoliators: Your calluses won't stand a chance!

no-fun bunions

Bunions, corns, and calluses are often referred to in the same breath, but they're very different things. A bunion occurs when the joint at the bottom of your big toe becomes inflamed— usually from wearing shoes that put a great amount of pressure on it, such as very high heels with pointed toes.

A bunion looks like a knob of bone sticking out from the side of your big toe, and can painfully push your big toe in toward the others. You can relieve pressure on bunions by wearing supportive shoes with nonconstricting toe boxes, or you can consult a medical professional about surgical options. (For information on calluses and corns, see pages 128 and 129.)

Avoid "corn plasters," medicated pads, and other over-the-counter corn treatments. They can cause severe irritation and discomfort. If your corns are particularly painful or are getting in the way of everyday life, see a medical professional rather than treating them yourself.

Infection Protection

Whenever we start talking to our clients about cleanliness and sanitation, the inevitable question arises: "How can I tell if I have an infection?" The first indication is probably a visual one: perhaps a change in the color, thickness, or texture of your toenails. If this sort of severe, sudden change appears, you need to contact a health professional. Fungal and bacterial infections, including athlete's foot, are highly contagious, so until you've got the all-clear from your doctor, you absolutely must not share nail-care implements, socks, towels, or shoes with anyone.

Think Thick

I have three "poodle toes"—thick, curved, slightly discolored nails—on my right foot that my dear dad passed along to me. If, like me, you've had this all your life, you have no choice but to file down and buff the top of the nail so it will be slightly thinner and flatter. Once buffed, you can treat the nail as normal, and every so often revisit it with the buffer to smooth down new growth.

If the thickening and discoloration have newly appeared, definitely contact a health professional to make sure nothing's infected.

My Feet Just Plain Stink

Foot sweat, like sweat anywhere else on you, is your body's way of staying cool. And part of the reason feet are *so* funky-smelling is that they're trapped inside our shoes all day, letting the sweat ferment into that familiar unpleasant odor. Keep your feet and shoes clean, and you should be able to avoid the worst odors.

Still, sometimes that's not enough. There are plenty of powders on the market that claim to eliminate foot odors, and some of them work quite well, but they're often quite expensive. A simple swipe of antiperspirant on the bottom of your foot can work miracles—just be sure to let it dry before slipping your feet into your shoes, or you'll be sliding around all day.

If you like things high-tech, talk to your doctor about prescription-strength products to limit perspiration and odor.

Oh My God, My Toenail Just Fell Off!

Toenails don't just fall off on a whim—there is no toenail fairy. If your toenail turns purple or starts lifting off, you probably injured it by dropping something on it, banging into something, slamming it in a door, or otherwise jamming the nail so hard that the matrix is disturbed. The purple color is likely a bruise forming under the nail (or it could be dried blood, if the skin on the nail bed split and bled), which your traumatized matrix root will decide either to let grow out or to give up on and grow a brand-new nail underneath. Let nature run its course—don't peel off the old nail until it's ready to go, and don't try to puncture or drain the bruise yourself. Cover it with a Band-Aid if it looks unsightly. While your new nail is growing in, go easy on your feet: Avoid tight-fitting shoes and high heels that put pressure on the big toe.

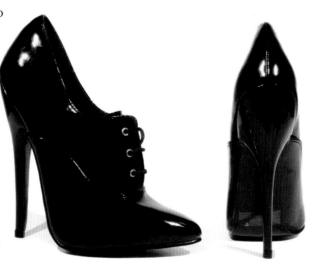

Some people—like me— would rather be taller. But shoes like these are no good for healthy feet.

If a bruised or falling-off toenail is causing you serious discomfort, see a doctor or another medical professional.

Athlete's Feet

If you're an athlete, particularly if your sport involves a lot of running, you probably know how embarrassing it can be to sit down in front of your pedicurist. Bruised toes, ingrown nails, blisters, and even athlete's foot (a common fungal infection) are prices you're willing to pay for being so committed to fitness, but there are ways to help offset the pain and suffering. Here are a few tips that will keep your tired tootsies in shape, too.

■ Having the appropriate footwear is absolutely essential to protecting your toes. Whatever sport you play, from basketball to long-distance running, make sure your shoes give you good support and are properly fitted.

There are ways to offset the pain and suffering.

■ Have more than one pair of sneakers to ensure that your feet won't be exposed to sweat and moisture lingering from the previous day's workout. Not only will you be more comfortable, but rotating your shoes will also greatly diminish your chances of getting athlete's foot. Powdering your feet with something simple like baby powder (or an antifungal powder) before slipping into your shoes also helps keep your feet less sweaty, making them less hospitable to fungus and bacteria.

■ Blisters are perhaps the worst side effect of being active. One nasty blister is enough to keep anyone off the treadmill for a few days, but popping them will only make them more uncomfortable, not to mention prone to infection. As mentioned for black-and-blue toenails, you must let nature take its course. Once new skin begins to grow over the raw interior part of the

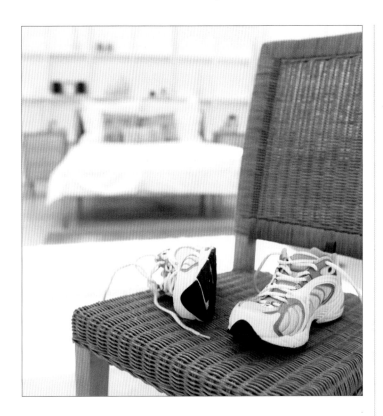

The proper shoes are as integral to your health as any other piece of equipment.

blister, the whole thing will deflate and the bubbled skin will peel away. In the meantime, soaking your feet in icy cold water will help soothe the pain and shrink the blisters, and lining problem areas of your shoes with moleskin can help prevent future ones from forming.

■ Keep your toenails short. As you run, your feet naturally slide forward in your shoes, so long toenails will be extra cramped. Trim and file regularly, and keep an eye out for ingrown nails— catching them early is the best way to train them back to normal.

■ If you do have ingrown nails, see the tips for treating them on page 127.

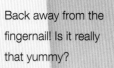

Back away from the
fingernail! Is it really
that yummy?

NBA (nail-biters anonymous)

Bad habits are like security blankets: They can be relaxing, they can calm your nerves, but at some point you just have to let them go.
And as far as bad habits go, nail-biting is up there in the hall of fame.
Everyone's been a nail-biter at one time or another—a nervous moment,
a day when you're too lazy to get the clipper, boredom at work.

Nail-biting is a way of life: Most biters' nails haven't seen a clipper or a file in years, their cuticles are nonexistent, and the damage to the matrix, or root, is severe. But whether you're a casual nibbler or a hard-core chomper, and no matter what your reason was for starting, now is the time to stop.

In my years at Rescue, what seems like thousands of nail-biters have come through the door. Many are dragged in by friends or family members who are sick and tired of their loved one's ragged-looking fingers; some come in of their own volition. They are all there to take advantage of what I call NBA—Nail-Biters Anonymous, my surefire twelve-week system for breaking yourself of the nail-biting habit.

If you're tired of dealing with your biting ways, salvation is here—no more hiding your hands. No more dreading a simple handshake. The tools for success are all in the next few pages.

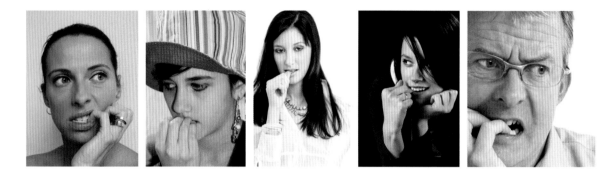

Biters come in all shapes, colors, ages, genders, and sizes.

Kicking the Habit

NBA began with a group of seven nail-biting clients who came in for a manicure every Sunday morning. Over base coat and cuticle oil, they helped each other through the process, sharing their nail-biting improvements and setbacks, and taking encouragement from one another. Now, almost a decade after this first meeting, all but one of the original participants still have gorgeous, healthy, unbitten nails. Based on their success, I've passed along the twelve-week technique—and emphasized the importance of finding support, in whatever form works for you—to clients of all ages, genders, and degrees of nail-biting severity.

While I've had an astonishing success rate with NBA, the most successful quitters—the ones who, years later, are still bite-free—are the ones who were truly committed to quitting. As with any bad habit, the first step in stopping is really *wanting* to stop. If the look of your bitten-to-the-quick nails isn't enough to motivate you to start breaking yourself of the nail-biting habit, stop and think: Biting your nails has more than just aesthetic consequences.

The nail's structure and growth operate not unlike a tree: The nail grows out from a root called the matrix and covers a specific area on the top of your finger known as the nail bed—the nail that covers it is called the nail plate (for a detailed diagram

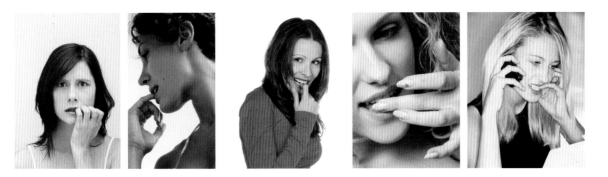

see page 10). When you bite your nails, you change the shape of your nail bed: The sides narrow as you pick and chew off hang-nails and bite off nail corners, and as you bite your nails lower and lower down your fingertip, the nail bed shortens, disturb-ing the matrix and affecting growth. Long-term nail-biters might notice that their nails are gnarled, lumpy, or irregularly colored. This effect is compounded by the fact that when your nail bed is so short, calluses begin to develop on the tips of your fingers as you rely on them more and more to replace the strength that your nails previously provided. Not unlike the calluses that form on the fingers of musi-cians, they—ironically—prevent your nail beds from returning to their original shape by blocking further outward nail growth.

Cuticle biting can inflict lasting damage as well: The folds of skin at the bottom and sides of your nail are living tissue, and their presence prevents moisture, bacteria, and other environ-mental toxins from getting underneath your nail plate and caus-ing damage. By biting or picking off your cuticles, you limit your skin's ability to protect the sensitive nail bed. Not to mention that heavy picking—which can produce scar tissue—amounts to "training" your cuticles not to grow back.

While I've had an astonishing success rate with NBA, the **most successful quitters** are the ones who were truly committed to quitting.

twelve weeks to a new you

save your teeth

Biting your nails doesn't just damage your fingers. You can also harm your teeth with the constant biting. It wears down the enamel, and increases the risk of chips and breaks. Do you really want to chip a tooth and have a hockey-player smile—from a habit as nonviolent as biting your nails?

Once you've made the decision to stop biting your nails, it's time to commit to healing. Of course, you won't grow perfect, beautiful nails overnight. It will take time to get your nails back to their healthy state, and to break yourself of the psychological impulse to put tooth to nail. I've found that a great way to start is with pen and paper: Write down three reasons you want to stop biting your nails. By committing it to writing, you're demonstrating that you take this decision seriously, and you're making it seem more real.

Once you've started implementing your decision to stop biting your nails, treat this project the way you'd treat any other project in your life: Set goals and deadlines. Get it into your head: every hour, day, or week without a bitten nail is a victory. View quitting as part of your daily routine: Get up in the morning and proudly declare, "I am not going to bite my nails today!"

No matter how firmly resolved you are about ending your nail-biting life, you still have to overcome the physical urge to chomp away. I've found that one of the best ways to do this is to redirect the impulse. Like a cigarette smoker chewing a piece of gum or an overeater going for a walk, you can get over nail-biting one incident at a time by just occupying your mind—and hands—with something else whenever you get the nibbling urge. My emergency kit (see page 140) is a great tool to set you on the path for success—couple it with the program outlined on page 142, and you're on your way!

male biters

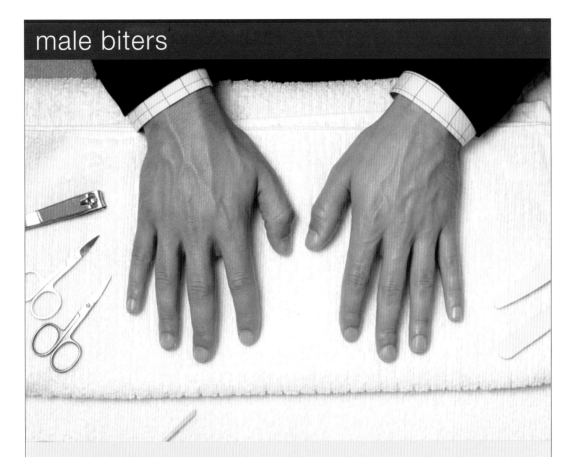

Any men out there who are undertaking NBA might be a little daunted by the idea of manicuring their nails once a week. While my older gentlemen clients are faithful about showing up for their buffs or coats of clear polish, not all guys are used to the idea of spa-style pampering for their hands. The truth is, there's no better way to get gorgeous nails than to dive right in to the joys of personal grooming. If you've never had a manicure before, you might want to get one professionally your first week (or more, if you like), to get a sense of how it's done. Just be sure to let the technician know that you're trying to get over a bad nail-biting habit, so she doesn't exacerbate it by trimming or filing too harshly.

If you're lucky, you might find a technician you really bond with, and she (or he) can be a real hands-on cheerleader to you through your twelve weeks of recovery.

the emergency kit

Those flaky bits of skin and nails might be calling to be chewed, but you can keep yourself in line with this simple emergency kit. Keep it nearby—in your handbag, in a desk drawer, in your glove compartment. If you see a hangnail or a jagged edge, or if you're just feeling the urge to bite, reach for something from your emergency kit to stop the problem in its tracks.

what you'll need

Cuticle cream (or eye cream, which is also nutrient-dense)

Small metal nail file or several disposable files

Small cuticle scissors

Hand sanitizer

Rubbing alcohol wipes

Neosporin

Ten Band-Aids

how to use your kit

■ Make a habit of regularly applying cuticle cream to your fingers. Not only does well-moisturized skin flake less easily (and less temptingly!) than dry skin, but the smell and taste of the cream will make your digits a little less appetizing.

■ Apply hand sanitizer frequently—it'll make the taste of your nails even more off-putting (though don't forget to moisturize to counterbalance the drying effects of the alcohol in the sanitizer).

■ If the corner of a nail is lifting or a chunk of side cuticle is flaking, take a deep breath and *do not pick*. Using the scissors from your emergency kit, trim the loose bit of nail or skin, and then use the file to smooth down the surrounding area.

■ If you know you're about to lose control and relapse to your biting ways, put Band-Aids on all your fingernails. Sure, it might look silly, but it's no more embarrassing than hiding your hands or walking around with bloody fingers.

■ If you slip up and bite your nail or cuticle so deeply that you're bleeding, clean the spot with a rubbing alcohol wipe, add a dab of Neosporin, and apply a Band-Aid.

Don't forget to regularly sterilize your metal implements (or replace disposable ones), and keep up your supply of Band-Aids, Neosporin, and hand sanitizer—don't wait until you've run out to refill your supplies. Treat your emergency kit as your first line of defense against the urge to bite, and you'll find success comes just that much more easily!

The emergency kit is your safety net—
keep it with you always.

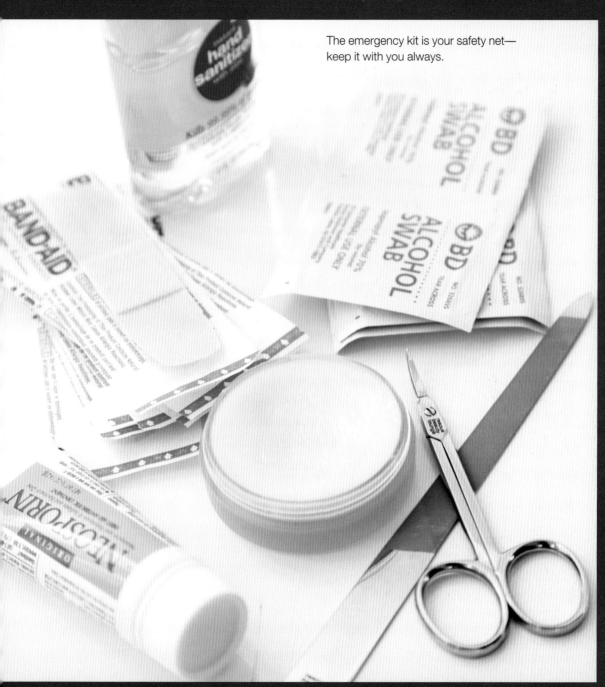

the program

mise en place

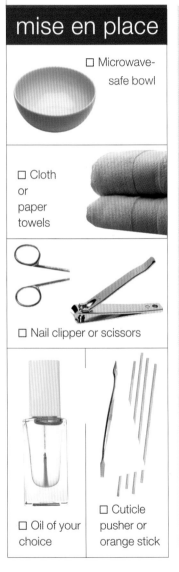

☐ Microwave-
safe bowl

☐ Cloth
or
paper
towels

☐ Nail clipper or scissors

☐ Oil of your
choice

☐ Cuticle
pusher or
orange stick

Besides your emergency kit and your deep reserves of willpower, you'll also need to set aside some time. But it's not much: just thirty minutes each week for the next twelve weeks. You'll use this time to give yourself a manicure (or, if you feel like it, get a professional one). Consider these 30-minute sessions serious, unbreakable commitments—write them on your calendar in ink!

Weeks 1-4

Boot Camp

Besides the simple willpower required to stop biting, it's been my experience that clients are less likely to bite their nails if the nails are well groomed and the cuticles are well moisturized. We're going to spend the first four weeks of your recovery getting your hands back to a good starting point, which requires intense hydration and diligent upkeep. The foundation for this is the Recovery Manicure (see facing page).

Over the course of these four weeks, the biggest change you'll see in your nails is simple: growth. It's possible that you might not know what to do with your new, longer nails. Be a little more careful during your everyday activities—digging your keys out of your bag or pocket, holding utensils, making phone calls. Be aware of how your nails affect the way you use your hands, and make sure you don't fall into any bad nail habits: You might notice that you're using your nails rather than your fingers to type, or that you're using them to button your shirt. It's natural to experience some clumsiness, and if your nails grow quickly and you find that they're interfering with your daily activities, feel free to gently file them down.

the recovery manicure

mise en place

Set yourself up with the tools and products listed on page 142.

step-by-step

1. Wash your hands with hot water and soap. Dry well.

2. Lay out terry-cloth or paper towels to prevent oil damage to your work area. Lay out your tools.

3. Fill the bowl halfway with the oil.

4. Warm the bowl of oil in the microwave for 10 seconds. (Microwave strengths vary, so be wary of getting the oil too hot—you want it to be warm to the touch, but not scalding. If the oil isn't warm enough after 10 seconds, warm it in 3-second increments, testing it with your fingertips at each interval.) Two or three times in rapid succession, dip the fingertips of one hand into the oil, coating your fingernails.

5. Dip that hand fully into the bowl of oil, and let it soak for one minute. Careful—dripping or spilled oil makes a mess! Be sure to have plenty of toweling on hand.

6. Once a minute has passed, remove your hand from the bowl and place it on a clean terry or paper towel. Holding your cuticle pusher in your other hand, gently push up the cuticles and around the nail bed of the oiled hand. There's probably a lot of dead skin around the cuticle—feel free to be a little aggressive in your pushing.

7. Repeat steps 5 and 6 on the same hand, reheating the oil in the microwave if necessary. In fact, you can repeat these two steps as many times as you like, until you're bored or you run out of dead skin to push away!

8. Once you're satisfied with your pushed-up cuticles, take the cuticle scissors in your unoiled hand and use them to trim off the excess skin. Take care to cut off only dead skin and not to cut into living tissue.

You might actually be able to see the half moon that was hidden.

9. Gently pat down your fingernails and skin—don't rub—with toweling to remove the excess oil.

10. Repeat the entire process on your other hand.

11. Go on to the At-Home Rescue Manicure, page 39. As tempted and inspired as you might be by this new beginning, now is not the time to be wearing nail polish. Your new growth needs to breathe, so just keep your hands clean and well cared-for—you'll be able to go wild with polish colors in the next phase.

During this initial period, make sure to moisturize your hands constantly. Not only will that help keep your nails and cuticles healthy, but you'll be less likely to want to put a hand that's covered with a perfumed emollient into your mouth.

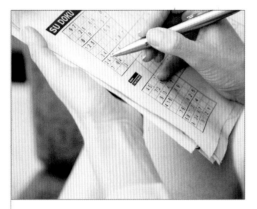

Also keep an eye out for new bad habits that replace your old ones. Some nail-biters turn into cuticle chewers, and vice versa.

The Recovery Manicure is similar to a basic manicure (page 39), but you'll be using one critical ingredient: oil. I would particularly recommend a natural essential oil that contains antibacterial agents: lemon, lime, orange, sage, rosemary, or arnica. Moroccan rose oil is another favorite of mine. But to be perfectly honest, essential oil can be pricey, and you're going to need a lot of it. So you can use any oil you like—commercial cuticle oil, vitamin E oil, olive oil, or corn oil, for example.

Weeks 5-8

Recovery

Congratulations! You've made it through an entire month without biting your nails . . . Right? By now, you've established your new routine: Once a week you spend thirty minutes tending to your fingers, and every day you make sure you're not biting, picking, or chewing at your cuticles or nails.

Each of these four weeks, you're still going to set aside that half hour for nail care: the recovery oil soak followed by a basic manicure. On top of maintaining the weekly nail care routine, you also must learn to perform your daily routines with your new nails. Now is the time for psychological vigilance: Your new, healthy, long nails and lush, hydrated cuticles are ripe for biting and picking. Don't! This is the make-or-break time in recovery!

Pay attention to the maintenance of your longer nails and healthy cuticles. Each week, during your manicure, pay attention to the shape and length of your nails. Try to maintain a healthy length that suits both your lifestyle and your aesthetics. This is also a good time to start introducing nail polish—it's not only attractive but has the added benefits of strengthening your nails and (on the off-chance you have a relapse and go in for a little nibble) tasting *awful.* Men can use clear polish. Women should stick to something pale and neutral—your nails still might be showing some irregularities from your old biting habits, and you don't want to call attention to that with a bright or dark color.

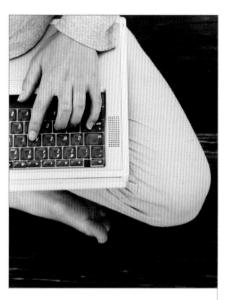

Of course, as always, you are your own best cheerleader. Keep positive about your progress, be vigilant with your emergency kit, and if you need to, repeat the recovery oil soak twice a week. You can never nurture your nails too much.

Moisturize regularly, file down any chips or tears, and as always—don't bite!

Weeks 9-12 — *The Promised Land*

We're almost done! From here on in, you can eliminate the recovery oil soak (unless you feel your nails really need the extra attention).

When you look at your hands now, you should see a real difference: longer, even nails that are couched in smooth, well-hydrated cuticles. Stick with your weekly maintenance to get yourself used to paying attention to your nails, and feel free to have some fun in the nail polish department: Bright, fun, outgoing colors are a perfect match for your new nails!

Thanks to your healthy fingernails, you just might find yourself in a better mood, a better humor, and—most important—feeling a whole lot more confident. Now work those nails. Flaunt them!

Once the Twelve Weeks Are Over

Congratulations! Now go back to page 38 to learn how to take care of your gorgeous, healthy nails.

Turning the file over
to a pro can be a
great way to relax.

professional nail service

As wonderful as an at-home manicure is, there are times when you just want to lean back and leave things to the professionals. But it's good to be informed: What should you look for in a spa? What's the etiquette for an awkward situation? How can you make your manicure last seemingly forever? The answers are all here.

t used to be that getting a manicure was a treat for a special occasion. We'd take time out of our busy lives to go to a high-end salon or fancy spa and sit in a quiet, soothing room while a nail technician buffed and massaged and polished us to perfection. But thanks to the proliferation of corner nail salons offering treatments for the same price as a workday lunch, manicures and pedicures can be a weekly or monthly indulgence for many of us.

Keep in mind, though, the prices at these corner salons are so low for a reason: The owners keep up their bottom line by cutting corners. Where once nail spas were about luxury, being pampered and catered to, they're now quick, impersonal models of efficiency—fifteen minutes from the first swipe of the nail polish remover to being whisked over to the drying station. And why shouldn't it be this way? Despite having the luxury stripped away, lower prices allow more

WARNING! whirlpool alert!

Pedicure whirlpool stations seem luxurious, don't they? But beware! They're actually incredibly unhygienic and dangerous. While most salons are good about rinsing and disinfecting the basins and faucets of the whirlpools, I dare you to ask your salon personnel when the last time was that they changed the filters in their whirlpool footbaths.

A whirlpool footbath runs all its water through a giant filter, so all sorts of bacteria, dirt, and debris get caught in there, including dead skin and clipped nails. The filter should be cleaned after each use, but I don't think I've ever seen that happen. Ask them to keep the jets off—or better yet, go to a salon that cares about sanitation and doesn't have whirlpool footbaths!

women (and men) to get regular salon manicures and pedicures than ever before.

Still, you get what you pay for. It's important to make sure that, as a client, you are getting the best possible service from your professional. You don't want to wind up somewhere that's not up to health and safety codes, or doesn't sterilize tools between clients. It's not necessary to go overboard, researching a particular salon's history with the board of health and the life stories of all the nail technicians. But you should treat a visit to a nail salon the same way you'd treat a visit to a new restaurant: Trust in word of mouth, make sure you feel comfortable, and—ultimately—trust your own judgment.

We all want a perfect, sterile, germ-free environment with perfectly trained and skilled technicians. But in our less-than-perfect world, we often have to accept that we can't always have that. When you go to a salon for the first time, there are things you'll want to make sure are in place. Use your common sense: The technicians should be licensed, there shouldn't be a pervasive chemical smell (this indicates that there isn't proper ventilation, which is particularly a problem if the salon applies acrylic nails), and work surfaces should be visibly clean. Last, but not at all least, you should feel welcomed and comfortable—this is an investment of your time and money, and you don't want to waste either one!

What to Look for in a Professional Salon

It's true that a spa manicure is a luxurious way to ensure that your nails look perfect, but the experience isn't all about the end result. You should go into your salon knowing what you hope to get out of your time and money: Do you want a relaxing experience? A cuticle tune-up? A perfect coat of polish? All three?

Whatever you're after, it all starts with your technician. It's important that you, as the client, be comfortable with the person

There's more to a
professional salon
manicure than just
the wall of polish.

my personal salon pet peeves

It happened to me!

■ *Seeing a technician use the same files and buffing blocks over and over again.*

■ *Salons that store their tools in medical pouches, but don't actually have an autoclave sterilizing their tools.*

■ *Technicians who use their own long nails to push a client's cuticles back—gross!*

■ *Salons that sell "personal" drawers for "your" tools. There's no way to know that those tools are being used only for you! (For more on this, see page 155)*

who is going to get up close and personal with your fingers and toes. You shouldn't be afraid to talk to her about what she's doing, or if there is a language barrier—as there often is—to ask the owners or other staff to translate for you.

When dealing with your technician, comfort can come in many guises. There are some visual clues to look for in a good manicurist: Her appearance should be neat and clean, she should be gentle and confident when handling her tools, and she shouldn't have long nails of her own, with the exception of a slightly longer thumb or pointer nail, which can be useful when applying polish (a technician who has long nails might sacrifice a perfect job on your nails in order to preserve her own). Your interaction with your technician should also be easy: She should never make you feel embarrassed about the state of your nails, or like you're a bad person for having an imperfect "canvas" for her to work on. She should be attentive to what *you* want, and able to take direction if you have specific requests or instructions.

Keep in mind that your technician is not a mind reader. Don't be shy about expressing your concerns and communicating your preferences. If your technician sneezes or coughs and then continues working without sanitizing his or her hands, don't hesitate to say, very nicely, "Would you mind washing your hands?" Don't say "Do whatever you think is best" unless you trust your technician completely, and know that she or he is clear about what results you expect. If you don't know precisely what you want, ask your technician about the various options available to you—the difference between pushing and cutting your cuticles, for example.

As in any relationship, both you and your technician will get frustrated if you can't communicate. What follows are some common client complaints, and my advice on the easiest way to handle the tricky technician/client relationship.

Q&A: spa and salon etiquette

What should I do if I become uncomfortable with my technician in the middle of my treatment?

If your technician does something that makes you uncomfortable, speak up! Tell her what's bothering you, and if she doesn't correct it, politely remove your hand or foot from her hold, excuse yourself from her station, go to the front desk, and ask to be switched to a new technician. Be specific about why you don't like the current one, so that the salon owners understand where you're coming from: "She's a bit rough and I'm really sensitive. Do you have anyone who is gentler?"

Don't just sit there and suffer through. You'll be hurting your technician's income by not tipping well, not to mention wasting your own time and money, and the bad mood that your unhappy salon experience is likely to cause won't do anybody any good. Communicate!

I don't think the place I frequent is clean enough, but I adore my technician. What should I do?

If you and your technician have a close relationship, be honest: Tell her that you think the place should be cleaner. If she doesn't want to lose you as a regular client, odds are good that she'll take your complaint higher up to the owners, and she'll also make sure that the salon—or at least her station—is spotlessly clean when you come for your next visit.

If you do mention something to your technician, but don't see any results, it's time to move on. Change is good. I'm sure there is another sweet technician (who does a great job) in a clean place.

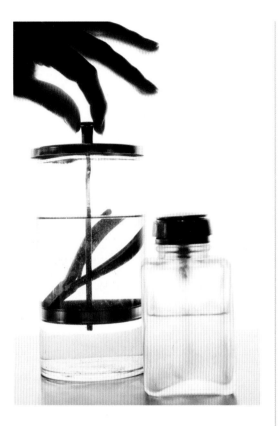

Can I ask the technician to clean the pedicure sink/ use a new set of tools/wash her hands before she begins working with me?

Yes! You can and you absolutely should. Your technician should go along with your request, and if she seems bothered by your desire for a more hygienic environment, it's

a good reason for you to leave immediately. My escape act is a quick glance at my watch, followed by "Oh no! I'm so sorry, I completely forgot that I'm supposed to meet a friend." This little white lie hurts no one, and it gets you out of that awful feeling of being trapped with a technician who isn't concerned with your health and hygiene.

What if I smudge my polish? Can I ask my technician to fix it?

This all depends on *when* you smudge your polish. If it's while the technician is still working on your hands (say you've been naughty and scratched your nose or used your cell phone), she should absolutely agree to fix it. Same goes if you're under the dryer and accidentally lift your hands too high. Even if you get a smudge while getting into your car once you've left the salon, just head back in immediately and apologetically (after all, you've ruined her artistic creation!) ask your technician to do a quick touch-up.

If it's been a few days and you chip your polish, there's often no need to get a whole new manicure. Call the salon and make an appointment to simply update your one or two chipped nails. Don't forget to tip for this, even if it's inexpensive—especially if your technician has made room in a busy schedule for you.

How much should I tip?

This varies from spa to spa and region to region, but a safe bet is—like a restaurant—between 15 and 20 percent of the total cost of your treatments. At a reputable spa, the entire tip goes to the technician, so don't be shy about giving her a due reward in exchange for her being knowledgeable, gentle, and responsive to your needs.

If you feel like your manicure was undeserving of a tip, don't do it! I might get hung out to dry for saying this, but you shouldn't ever feel *obligated* to tip your technician. It's a gesture of thanks given after the fact. If your salon tries to make you pay and tip before the polish is even on and you'd rather wait to see the outcome of the manicure, simply ask kindly if you can take care of the transaction once the service is done.

My experience was awful— I just wanted to get up and leave!

Speak up! Every business ultimately wants satisfied clients, and sometimes it's hard to make the tastes and techniques of the client match perfectly with those of the techinician. Make sure you say something before it's too late: Give the technician, or the salon, a chance to fix the mistake.

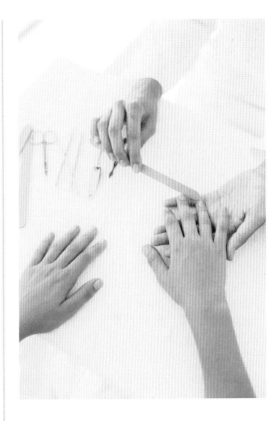

Don't worry about hurting the technician's feelings if things get really out of hand and you're being physically harmed or your boundaries are being violated. Stop the procedure immediately and ask for help from the manager, owner, or another attendant.

sanitation and sterilization

taking your own tools to the salon

If you have your own set of nail care tools, and they're clean and well maintained, by all means take them with you to the salon! But, really, make sure they're clean and well maintained. You wouldn't believe some of the sets my clients bring to me—I want to cringe and put on gloves before even touching them. Use only metal tools that are dirt- and debris-free, and that have been sterilized beforehand: See page 36 for details on how to sterilize your tools.

Unlike a haircut or a massage, nail care treatments often verge on being medical: In the course of a manicure, you'll be snipped and cut and scraped and filed, and your delicate skin can run the risk of being exposed to any number of nasty things. Without proper sanitation and sterilization, you run the risk of a bacterial or fungal infection being transmitted to you via tools, surfaces, or even your technician's hands. To help offset this risk, all nail salons are required by law to abide by strict sterilization codes, especially when it comes to tools. There are a number of methods by which they can go about it.

One of the most common sterilization methods is to use an **ultraviolet ray box** that looks like a toaster oven. On the upside, most salons have access to these because they aren't too expensive. On the downside, the tools need a full 25 to 30 minutes in the box before they're fully sterilized—*and* they have to be laid out flat, not stacked on top of each other. This becomes an almost unattainable goal at most salons during busy times with high client turnover.

Good old-fashioned **liquid disinfectant,** an ammonia-based substance often found under the brand name Barbicide, is another way to get tools free of germs. The liquid should be kept in a clear, airtight container, and should be clear blue or pink and free of any floating particles. Like the UV box, Barbicide also takes about 25 minutes to fully clean the tools of all bacteria. Ideally, each technician should have two jars, so that one set of tools can be getting sterilized while the other is in use. And, naturally, the solution should be changed whenever it's cloudy, ideally at least once a day.

The most efficient and foolproof method of sterilization is the **autoclave.** This machine really is my true love. It's the machine used by hospitals and dentists to ensure the highest degree of sterility of their tools. It works by heating metal tools to an extremely high temperature using a built-in timer and thermometer, in an environment completely free of moisture. It can't be opened during the sterilization process.

Sterilization doesn't stop once the germs are dead, however. If your technician isn't going to use the tools immediately after they are sterilized, the method of storing them is as important as the initial sterilization. Tools must be sealed in individual airtight pouches, so after all that work that was done to kill the old germs, they aren't exposed to new ones borne by air and surface dirt.

The Three S's: Sanitation, Sterilization, and Storage

There is no such thing as an entirely germ-free environment, but it's helpful to know what you should look out for. At Rescue Beauty Lounge, we ask a sneaky question on our employee application: "What is the difference between sanitation and sterilization?" In order to pass the exam to get a nail technician's license, you need to know this—but you wouldn't believe the answers we get.

Sanitation means to make something clean: keeping all surfaces free of debris, dust, and dirt. All nail technicians need to sanitize their workstations, but that's not enough.

Sterilization means to make something free of bacteria and other microorganisms, and applies to all metal tools and implements.

Storage is the third *S,* and it's just as important. It should always be airtight—a Ziploc bag or a medical pouch is a good sign.

storing your tools at the salon

For a few dollars, many professional salons will offer a personal set of tools that they'll happily store for you on the premises. I'm sure this is relaxing knowledge to some people, but it would drive me crazy—how do you know how often they clean your tools, sterilize the metal, or replace the disposable elements? Even if you trust that your tools will be used only on you, there's still a risk of infection: Just because you're the only user, it doesn't mean germs won't breed and grow. It's better to keep your own set at home, where you can control the cleanliness level, and take your tools into the salon when it's time for a touch-up.

demystifying the manicure

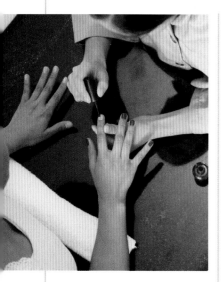

Every salon manicure should conform to a basic outline of services and techniques. While spas and technicians might vary slightly in what tools they use or in the type of massage they give, you're missing out if your manicure and pedicure don't contain these basic elements.

Removing Old Polish

This gives the technician a clean canvas to work on. Even if you're not wearing any polish, you still might get a swipe of polish remover, since it removes any oils and dirt that might have built up on the surface of the nail.

Filing and Buffing

The nail file and the buffing block come next, and are used to even the length and smooth the surface of your nails. If you're shortening your nails by any significant degree, this is when it should happen: Tell your technician you'd like your nails short, and she'll take out the clippers or the rough-grade file. Buffing seals the top of your nail, further smoothing the surface for the eventual application of polish.

Soaking and Cuticle Care

This is the real meat of the manicure. Once your nails are trimmed and buffed, you'll soak them for a few minutes in a solution of warm, soapy water. This loosens the skin of your cuticles, which helps the technician push or trim them away. Working first with one hand or foot, and then the other, your technician will cut or push your cuticles off the nail plates, and then resubmerge the hand or foot in the soapy water.

Exfoliation, Moisturization, and Massage

Once the cuticles are taken care of, attention shifts to the whole hand. Your skin should be scrubbed with an exfoliating cream or cleanser, rinsed thoroughly (often followed by a warm towel), and then comes the part that my clients love: Moisturizer of some sort—lotion, cream, or oil—is massaged into the skin with firm, relaxing, circulation-improving strokes.

The Icing on the Cake: Polish

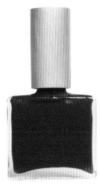

After your technician removes any oily residue from the moisturizing massage, she'll apply base coat, a coat or two of color, and the topcoat. The polish is the pretty part, but the real heart of the manicure is everything that came before.

Drying Time

You should be given plenty of time to allow your newly polished nails to dry. Never let yourself be rushed out the door! Whether it's under UV lights, a fan, or simple air-drying (my preferred method), your manicure will be at its best if you take this time to let the polish fully harden. Give yourself at least 15 minutes—20 if you can afford it. The longer, the better.

keep it up!

at-home maintenance

A salon manicure can be expected to last, at most, six days, and a pedicure will last twenty. When I'm asked by clients how often they should come in for treatments, though, I tell them to come in once a week for their hands, and twice a month for their toes. Why is that? It's because—as I've explained through this chapter—the manicure is a lot more than just the shiny, colorful polish. While a well-done polish application should last for seven to ten days, your cuticles and skin are best served with weekly and fortnightly maintenance updates.

But a ten-day manicure is still only a best-case scenario. Most barely last five. What can you do to prolong that beautiful, glossy finish? Use common sense, mostly. Here are some tips to help you along the way.

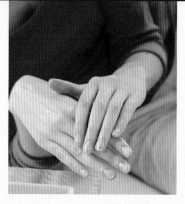

at the salon

■ Have your payment, car keys or cab fare, and house keys out and ready before the polish goes on. But remember—if possible, don't pay or tip until after the manicure is over and you're satisfied with the results.

■ Don't dig through your purse for anything—the hairband can wait, no matter how huge the hair emergency!

■ Ask someone to open the door for you when you leave.

once manicured

■ Don't shower, if possible, for about six hours after your manicure. If you must shower, don't use very hot water. The heat of the water will soften your laquer, opening the possibility of its melting into that annoying smush at the tip.

■ Don't take a nap. Who knows what you do with your hands while you sleep! You certainly don't want to get polish all over your sheets—or have sheet marks on your polish!

every day until you take the polish off

■ Moisturize. Always.

■ Apply a new layer of topcoat every other day. Not only does this reinvigorate the shine on your nails, but it's insurance against chips and smudges.

■ Don't use your nails as tools! Most chips happen at the tip, and they'll be hurried along if you use your fingernails as can openers, screwdrivers, scrapers, and scratchers.

index

photo credits

Cover: Deborah Ory

Interior:

Original Photography by **Deborah Ory:** pages vi all, vii top, x, 14 all, 18, 21, 23 left, 25 top left, 27, 37, 38, 42, 45, 46, 51–56, 60–68, 71, 72, 76, 79 all, 80, 82, 87 all, 88–89, 90 top right, 100–2, 105 all except bottom right, 109, 111, 112, 117, 118, 121, 141, 158; **Jenna Bascom:** pages 4 second from left, 28–29 all, 30 top and middle, 31–33 all, 34 top, 35 all, 40 all, 58 all, 75 orange sticks and all nail polish bottles, 90 bottom right, 91–96 all, 124, 129, 142 scissors, clippers, cuticle pusher, and sticks, 157; **Katherine Gulick:** pages 5 far right, 30 bottom, 90 bottom left.

Stock Photography by **age fotostock:** Steve Wisbauer page 116; **Bridgeman Art Library:** page 4 far left; **Everett Collection:** pages 8 and 15; **Getty Images:** Greg Ceo page 4 far right, Hulton Archive page 5 far left, Nina Leen page 5 second from left, Chris Walter page 5 third from left, Graeme Montgomery page 5 fourth from left, Julie Toy page 26, Heidi Coppock-Beard page 70, Paul Tearle page 86, Jamie Grill page 90 top left, Pando Hall pages vii second from top, 107, and 134, Jeffrey Coolidge page 108, Steve Wisbauer page 116, ML Harris page 127, Stockbyte page 133, Grove Pashley pages vii fourth from top middle, 137 far left, Juan Silva page 137 second from left, Donata Pizzi pages vii fourth from top far right, 137 far right, Nicola Tree page 139, Dylan Ellis page 144 top, Lisa M. Robinson page 145, George Doyle pages vii bottom, 146, UpperCut Images page 149, Somos page 152; **iStockPhoto:** pages 23 and 113, Brian McEntire page 24 left, Johanna Goodyear page 24 right, Lei Leng Yiap pages 25 middle bottom, 41 products lower right, 59 products lower right, 99 lower right, Eric Hood pages 34 third from top, 41 supplies bottom left, 59 supplies middle left, 142 second from top, Emil Marinsek page 105 bottom right, Delphine Mayeur page 142 bottom left; **Mary Evans Picture Library:** page 4 third from left; **Punchstock:** Stockbyte page 153; **Shutterstock:** David Touchtone page 4 fourth from left, Domenico Gelermo page 16, s-dmit page 24 middle, Ewa Brozek pages 25 top right, 41 supplies top left, 59 supplies top left, 75 top left, 99 supplies middle left, Nat Ulrich pages 34 second from top, 59 bottom right, Stillfx pages 34 bottom, 41 top right, 59 top right, 7 lower left, 99 middle right, Travis Manley pages 41 top left, 59 top left, 74 products top left, 99 bottom left, Olga Lyubkina pages 41 bottom left, 59 bottom left, Scott Rothstein pages 41 products top right, 59 products top right, Angelo Girardelli pages 41 supplies bottom right, 142 top, RJ Lerich pages 59 middle right, 7 middle right, Maxstockphoto page 99 top, Feng Yu page 115, Terrence Mendoza page 131, mmm page 136 far left, Lori Carpenter page 136 second from left, Lev Dolgachov page 136 third from left, Domen Colja page 136 fourth from left, Peter Close pages vii fourth from top far left, 136 far right, Lev Olkha page 137 third from left, Wallenrock page 137 fourth from left; **Superstock:** page 58 cuticle scissors; **Veer:** page: 156 Blend Images Photography.